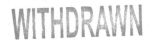

ERRATA

The National Diet and Nutrition Survey: adults aged 19 to 64 years.
Volume 1: Types and quantities of foods consumed.
Henderson L, Gregory J, Swan G. TSO (London, 2002).

WITHDRAWN

ISBN   0 11 621566 6

Since its publication in December 2002, an error has come to light in the derivation of consumption data for the following food types:

> Other cereals
> Cream
> Other milk
> Beef, veal & dishes
> Table sugar
> Fruit juice
> Concentrated soft drinks - not low calorie, as consumed
> Concentrated soft drinks - low calorie, as consumed
> Coffee, as consumed
> Tea, as consumed
> Other beverages, dry weight
> Soup

The following tables have been revised to show correct consumption figures and are available at www.food.gov.uk/science/:

> Tables 2.10(a) and 2.10(b); Tables 2.11(a), 2.11(b) and 2.11(c)
> Tables 2.12(a) and 2.12(b); Tables 2.13(a) and 2.13(b)
> Table 2.14; Table 2.16(b); Table 2.17(b)
> Tables A2(a), A3(a), A4(a), A5(a), A6(a), A7(a) and A8.

Data on nutrient intakes are not affected by this error.

The National Diet and Nutrition Survey: young people aged 4 to 18 years.
Volume 1: Report of the diet and nutrition survey.
Gregory JR, Lowe S, Bates CJ, Prentice A, Jackson LV, Smithers G, Wenlock R, Farron M. TSO (London, 2000).

ISBN   0 11 621265 9

The error noted above affects the consumption data for the following food types for the NDNS of young people aged 4 to 18 years:
> Whole milk
> Cream
> Other milk
> Concentrated soft drinks - not low calorie, as consumed
> Concentrated soft drinks - low calorie, as consumed
> Coffee, as consumed
> Tea, as consumed
> Other beverages, dry weight

Revised consumption figures for these food types are available at www.food.gov.uk/science/.

continued over

The National Diet and Nutrition Survey: adults aged 19 to 64 years.
Volume 2: Energy, protein, carbohydrate, fat and alcohol intake.
Henderson L, Gregory J, Irving K, Swan G. TSO (London, 2003).

ISBN   0 11 621567 4

CORRECTIONS

Page 9, section 2.2, para 1, second and third sentences to read:
'The mean daily total energy intake for men was 9.72MJ (2313kcal) and for women, 6.87MJ (1632kcal) ($p < 0.01$). Mean intake for men was significantly higher than for women in all age groups ($p < 0.01$).

Page 9, section 2.2, para 3, second and third sentences to read:
'The mean daily food energy intake for men was 8.88MJ (2110kcal) and for women, 6.54MJ (1554kcal) ($p < 0.01$). Mean intake for men was significantly higher than for women in all age groups ($p < 0.01$).

The National Diet and Nutrition Survey: adults aged 19 to 64 years.
Volume 3: Vitamin and mineral intake and urinary analytes.
Henderson L, Irving K, Gregory J, Bates CJ, Prentice A, Perks J, Swan G, Farron M. TSO (London, 2003).

ISBN   0 11 621568 2

CORRECTIONS

Page 12, section 2.2.1 Pre-formed retinol:
For 'mg' read 'μg'.

Page 17, section 2.3.7, para 2, first sentence:
For '41mg for men' read '41μg for men'.

Page 17, section 2.3.7, para 6, second sentence:
For 'within the range 10mg to 200mg' read 'within the range 10μg to 200μg'.

Page 40, Table 2.20
For percentage contribution of 'cheese' to average daily intake of niacin equivalents for men aged 19-24 years read '2', aged 25-34 years '2', aged 35-49 years '2', aged 50-64 years '3' and for all men '2'; for women aged 19-24 years read '2', aged 25-34 years '3', aged 35-49 years '2', aged 50-64 years '3' and for all women '2', for all respondents read '2'.

Page 52, Table 2.32:
For mean average daily intake of vitamin C (mg) from all sources for women aged 50-64 years read '128.0' and for all women read '112.4'.
For upper 2.5 percentile of average daily intake of vitamin C (mg) from all sources for women aged 50-64 years read '608.3'.
For standard deviation of average daily intake of vitamin C (mg) from all sources for women aged 50-64 years read '166.72' and for all women read '209.86'.

Page 53, Table 2.33:
For mean average daily intake of vitamin C (mg) as % of RNI from all sources for women aged 50-64 years read '320' and for all women read '281'.
For standard deviation of average daily intake of vitamin C (mg) as % of RNI from all sources for women aged 50-64 years read '416.8' and for all women read '524.6'.

Office for National Statistics
December 2004

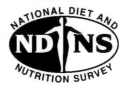

Volume 5

The National Diet & Nutrition Survey: adults aged 19 to 64 years

Summary Report

Jacqueline Hoare
Lynne Henderson
Office for National Statistics

with **Christopher J Bates**
Ann Prentice
Maureen Birch
*Medical Research Council
Human Nutrition Research*

Gillian Swan
Melanie Farron
Food Standards Agency

A survey carried out in Great Britain on behalf of the Food Standards Agency and the Departments of Health by the Office for National Statistics and Medical Research Council Human Nutrition Research

London: TSO

Contact points

For enquiries about this publication, contact
Jacqueline Hoare
Tel: 020 7533 5383
E-mail: jacqueline.hoare@ons.gsi.gov.uk

For general enquiries, contact the National Statistics Customer Contact Centre on: 0845 601 3034
(minicom: 01633 812399)
E-mail: info@statistics.gsi.gov.uk
Fax: 01633 652747
Post: Room 1015, Government Buildings,
Cardiff Road, Newport NP10 8XG

You can also find National Statistics on the Internet at:
www.statistics.gov.uk

About the Office for National Statistics

The Office for National Statistics (ONS) is the government agency responsible for compiling, analysing and disseminating many of the United Kingdom's economic, social and demographic statistics, including the retail prices index, trade figures and labour market data, as well as the periodic census of the population and health statistics. It is also the agency that administers the statutory registration of births, marriages and deaths in England and Wales. The Director of ONS is also the National Statistician and the Registrar General for England and Wales.

A National Statistics publication

National Statistics are produced to high professional standards set out in the National Statistics Code of Practice. They undergo regular quality assurance reviews to ensure that they meet customer needs. They are produced free from any political influence.

This report is dedicated to the memory of Jan Gregory (Ingram), the NDNS Programme Manager at ONS. Jan died unexpectedly in February 2004 before she could see this final volume published. Jan had a long professional association with the NDNS Programme and her expertise and personal interest in the subject contributed enormously to the scientific value of the series. Jan is sadly missed by all those involved.

Contents

Foreword

This survey, of a national sample of adults aged 19–64 years, is one of a programme of national surveys with the aim of gathering information about the dietary habits and nutritional status of the British population. The results of the survey will be used to develop nutrition policy and to contribute to the evidence base for Government advice on healthy eating.

This report, the fifth and final in a series covering this survey, summarises the key findings from the first four reports. The first report, covering foods consumed, was published in December 2002. The second, covering intakes of energy and macronutrients, and the third, covering vitamin and mineral intakes and urinary analytes, were published in July 2003. The fourth report covering physical measurements, blood pressure, physical activity levels, and a range of biochemical indices of nutritional status derived from analysis of blood samples, was published in February 2004.

The work described in this series of reports results from a successful collaboration between the Food Standards Agency and the Department of Health, who jointly funded the collection of the survey data, with the Office for National Statistics and the Medical Research Council Human Nutrition Research.

We warmly welcome this final report of the latest survey in the National Diet and Nutrition Survey programme and express our thanks to all the respondents who took part.

Sir John Krebs
Chairman
Food Standards Agency

Melanie Johnson
Minister for Public Health
Department of Health

Authors' Acknowledgements

We would like to thank everyone who contributed to the survey and the production of this report:

- the respondents without whose co-operation the survey would not have been possible;

- the ONS interviewers who recruited the respondents and carried out all the fieldwork stages of the survey;

- ONS colleagues in the Sampling Implementation Unit, Field Branch, Business Solutions, Methodology Unit and Project Support Branch, in particular, Amanda Wilmot, Jo Bacon, Dave Ruston, Bev Botting, Goli Lashkari, Ann Whitby, Michaela Pink, Karen Irving, Caroline Ojemuyiwa, Michael Staley, Glenn Edy, Andrew Tollington, Dave Elliot, Jeremy Barton and Tracie Goodfellow;

- the ONS nutritionists, namely Debbie Hartwell, Michaela Davies, Sui Yip, Laura Hopkins, Jessica Ive, Sarah Oyston, Claire Jaggers and Robert Anderson;

- the ONS editors, namely Angela Harris, Carole Austen, Mike Donovan, Nina Hall, Sue Heneghan, Sarah Kelly, Dave Philpot, Colin Wakeley, Carol Willis and Heather Yates;

- staff of the Medical Research Council Human Nutrition Research (HNR), particularly staff of the Micronutrient Status Laboratory, namely: Steve Austin, Shailja Nigdikar, Filomena Liuni, Karen Giddens, Hanneke Schippers, Neal Matthews, Glynn Harvey, Laura Wang, Richard Carter, Helen Martindale, Clare Kitchener, Jason Swain; and staff of the Survey Office, namely: Jolieke van der Pols, Robert Quigley, Roberta Re, Lucy Winter, Elaine Proud, Carmen Treacy, Kathleen Edwards, Gemma Bramwell, Michael Garratt, Ansar Malik, Dr Andy Coward and Dr Jayne Perks;

- the phlebotomists and local laboratory personnel who were recruited by HNR to take the blood samples, and process and store the blood specimens;

- Professor Elaine Gunter, Chief, National Health and Nutrition Examination Survey (NHANES) Laboratory, Centres for Disease Control and Prevention, Atlanta, USA, for an independent review of the methodology for the blood and urine sample collection and laboratory analyses;

- Professor Angus Walls for his contribution to the oral health component and briefing the interviewers on the procedures for the self-tooth and amalgam-filling count;

- Professor Chris Skinner and Dr David Holmes at the University of Southampton for an independent review of response to this NDNS and an assessment of non-response bias;

- David Marker at Westat for an independent review of NDNS methodology and procedures;

- the professional staff at the Food Standards Agency and the Department of Health, in particular Jamie Blackshaw, Mark Bush, Susan Church, Michael Day, Rebecca Finnamore, Miguel Goncalves, Hannah Green, Lynda Harrop, Tom Murray, John Pascoe, Dr Roger Skinner and Alette Weaver of the Food Standards Agency; Richard Bond, Tony Boucher, Ian Cooper, Dr Sheela Reddy and Robert Wenlock of the Department of Health.

Notes to the tables

Tables showing percentages

In general, percentages are shown if the base is 30 or more. Where a base number is less than 30, actual numbers are shown within square brackets.

The row or column percentages may add to 99% or 101% because of rounding and weighting.

The varying positions of the bases in the tables denote the presentation of different types of information. Where the base is at the foot of the table, the whole distribution is presented and the individual percentages add to between 99% and 101%. Where the base is given in a column, the figures refer to the proportion of respondents who had the attribute being discussed, and the complementary proportion, to add to 100%, is not shown in the table.

In tables showing cumulative percentages the row labelled 'All' is always shown as 100%. The proportion of cases falling above the upper limit of the previous band can be calculated by subtracting from 100 the proportion in the previous band. Actual maximum values are not shown in tables of cumulative percentages, since they could vary for different subgroups being considered within the same tables.

Unless shown as a separate group, or stated in the text or a footnote to a table, estimates have been calculated for the total number of respondents in the subgroup, excluding those not answering. Base numbers shown in the tables are the total number of respondents in the subgroup, including those not answering.

The total column may include cases from small subgroups not shown separately elsewhere on the tables, therefore the individual column bases may not add to the base in the total column.

Where categories presented in this Volume represent an amalgamation of categories shown in previous volumes, all percentages have been recalculated for the new category. Therefore, small differences, due to rounding, may exist between percentage values shown in tables in this Volume compared with values that could be calculated from previous volumes, for example, by summing percentages across categories.

Conventions

The following conventions have been used in the tables:

..	data not available
-	category not applicable; no cases
0	values less than 0.5%
[ ]	numbers inside square brackets are the actual numbers of cases, when the base is fewer than 30.

Tables showing descriptive statistics – mean, standard deviation

These are shown in tables to an appropriate number of decimal places.

Significant differences

Differences commented on in the text are those that have been found to be significant at the 95% or 99% confidence levels ($p<0.05$ and $p<0.01$). *See* Appendix C.

As a general indication of those groups showing the largest differences, the difference between all pairs of groups were tested for statistical significance. Because of this 'trawling' approach, real statistical significance levels are lower than indicated here and some of the reported significant differences are likely to be spurious. However, these significance tests can still be validly used for testing hypotheses suggested by earlier work.

Standard deviations

Standard deviations for estimates of mean values are shown in tables and have been calculated
for a simple random sample design. In testing for the significant difference between two estimates,
proportions or means, the sampling error calculated as for a simple random design was multiplied by
an assumed design factor of 1.5 to allow for the complex sample design (*see* Appendix C). In general,
design factors were below 1.5. Therefore although not commented on in the text, there will be some
differences in sample proportions and means, that are significantly different.

Weighting

Unless otherwise stated, all proportions and means presented in the tables in the substantive chapters
in this Volume are taken from data weighted to compensate for the differential probabilities of selection
and non-response. Base numbers are presented weighted. All base numbers are given in italics. *See*
Appendix B for further details on the weighting and for unweighted base numbers.

1 Background

This Volume presents summary findings on food and nutrient intake, physical measurements, nutritional status and physical activity from a survey of the diet and nutrition of adults aged 19 to 64 years living in private households in Great Britain, carried out between July 2000 and June 2001. It is the final volume in a series of five which provide key information relating to:

- foods consumed and nutrient intake;

- nutritional status (based on physical measurements amd analysis of blood samples);

- blood pressure; and

- physical activity.

The previous four volumes can be found on the Food Standards Agency website (www.food.gov.uk)[1].

This Volume presents key findings from the National Diet and Nutrition Survey (NDNS) of adults aged 19 to 64 years, highlighting areas of public and policy interest. More specifically, this Volume covers the following subjects:

- summary of foods consumed;

- portions of fruit and vegetables consumed;

- summary of nutrient intake with comparison to Dietary Reference Values;

- main food sources of key nutrients;

- intakes of salt;

- alcohol consumption;

- nutritional status (based on physical measurements and the analysis of blood samples);

- blood pressure; and

- physical activity levels.

Summary findings are presented by sex, age, region[2] and household receipt of benefits[3] and, where guidelines exist, data are compared against these. Also, where possible, data from this survey are compared to results from the Dietary and Nutritional Survey of British Adults aged 16 to 64 years, the last survey of this age group to be carried out (1986/87 Adults Survey)[4].

1.1 The National Diet and Nutrition Survey programme

This survey forms part of the National Diet and Nutrition Survey programme. This was set up jointly by the Ministry of Agriculture, Fisheries and Food (MAFF)[5] and the Department of Health. MAFF's responsibility for the NDNS Programme has now transferred to the Food Standards Agency. Previous surveys have covered other age groups within the population, namely older adults, pre-school children and young people[6,7,8]. The last national survey of diet and nutrition in adults was the 1986/87 Adults Survey[4].

The NDNS programme aims to provide comprehensive information on the dietary habits and nutritional status of the population of Great Britain. The results of all the surveys within the programme are used to develop nutrition policy at a national and local level, and to contribute to the evidence base for Government advice on healthy eating. For example, recent NDNS surveys have highlighted concern regarding high salt intakes and low consumption of fruit and vegetables in the population. For more information on the NDNS programme *see* Chapter 1 of the Technical Report[9].

1.2 The NDNS of Adults

Adults aged 19 to 64 years living in private households were selected at random to take part in this survey (for more information on sample design and selection, *see* Appendix A). The survey was carried out over a 12-month period, July 2000 to June 2001, to allow for differences in eating behaviour and the nutrient content of food (e.g. milk) between the different seasons. A Technical Report which contains all the methodology chapters and corresponding appendices relating to this NDNS is available online[9].

A feasibility study was carried out between September and December 1999 to test all components of this survey and suggest recommendations for revisions to the main survey (*see* Appendix C of the Technical Report[9]).

Following publication of this Volume, the full data set will be deposited with The Data Archive at the University of Essex[10].

1.3 The components of the survey

The survey includes various components in order to obtain the wide range of information required[11]. All respondents were eligible to take part in all components, but not all chose to participate in each one. Response rates to the different components are presented in Appendix B.

- Dietary interview

Initially a face-to-face dietary interview was carried out with the household member selected to take part in the survey (the respondent), to provide information about their eating and drinking habits, their socio-demographic circumstances (e.g. age and marital status) and the socio-demographic circumstances of their household (e.g. benefit status). The interview questionnaire is reproduced in Appendix A of the Technical Report[9].

- Seven-day weighed intake dietary record

Respondents were also invited to complete a dietary record for seven days. This involved weighing and recording all food and drink consumed both at home and away from home, including medicines taken by mouth and drinks of water. The dietary record collected detailed information in order to look at the range of food consumption and nutrient intake within the population. Food and nutrient intake data could also be related to physical activity and various nutritional status and health measures. *See* Appendix A of the Technical Report for the dietary record, and Appendix F of the Technical Report for a discussion of this methodology[9].

- 24-hour urine collection

Respondents were asked to carry out a 24-hour urine collection (*see* Appendix K of the Technical Report[9]). Samples taken from the collection were tested for a number of analytes and provided estimates of sodium (salt) intake[12].

- Physical measurements

Respondents could have height and weight measurements taken, and these were used to calculate Body Mass Index, which is a measure of 'fatness'. Waist and hip circumferences were also measured as these provide information on distribution of body fat and health status[13]. Blood pressure measurements were taken since high blood pressure is an important and known risk factor for cardiovascular disease in adults. Trained interviewers from the Office for National Statistics (ONS) took all these measurements within the respondent's home. The protocols for taking these measurements can be found in Appendix J of the Technical Report[9].

- Seven-day physical activity record

Data were also collected on physical activity, to allow an investigation of the relationships between dietary intakes, body composition and physical activity levels. Respondents were asked to record their physical activity over the same seven days as the dietary record was completed. The diary asked for details of time spent on a list of specified activities, and information was collected on duration and intensity of each of these activities. For more details on the physical activity component, *see* Appendix I of the Technical Report[9], and Appendix D of Volume 4[1].

- Blood sample

Blood samples were taken from consenting respondents and were analysed for a range of indicators which reflect the levels of certain nutrients available for use in the body. These included indicators for iron, vitamin C and cholesterol levels for example. All procedures associated with obtaining and analysing the blood samples were contracted to the Medical Research Council Human Nutrition Research (HNR) who are experts in this area. For more information on the procedures for this component *see* Appendix N and Appendix O of the Technical Report[9].

Due to the invasive aspects of some components of the National Diet and Nutrition Survey, it was essential to gain ethics committee approval before the survey could take place. Ethics committee approval was gained for both the feasibility and main survey from a Multi-centre Research Ethics Committee and National Health Service Local Research Ethics Committees as required (*see* Appendix N of the Technical Report[9]).

1.4 Response to the survey

Overall, 2,251 respondents completed the dietary interview. Of these, 1,724 also completed a full seven-day dietary record. As not everyone who was selected took part in the survey, there was a chance that data would be biased for different age and sex groups, so the data presented in this and other volumes are weighted to represent the general population. For full details on response to this survey, the different components, and how the survey was weighted, *see* Appendix B.

References and endnotes

1   The other volumes in this series are:

   (i) Henderson L, Gregory J, Swan G. *National Diet and Nutrition Survey: adults aged 19 to 64 years. Volume 1: Types and quantities of foods consumed.* TSO (London, 2002);

   (ii) Henderson L, Gregory J, Irving K, Swan G. N*ational Diet and Nutrition Survey: adults aged 19 to 64 years. Volume 2: Energy, protein, carbohydrate, fat and alcohol intake.* TSO (London, 2003);

   (iii) Henderson L, Irving K, Gregory J, Bates CJ, Prentice A, Perks J, Swan G, Farron M. *National Diet and Nutrition Survey: adults aged 19 to 64 years. Volume 3: Vitamin and mineral intake and urinary analytes.* TSO (London, 2003);

   (iv) Ruston D, Hoare J, Henderson L, Gregory J, Bates CJ, Prentice A, Birch M, Swan G, Farron M. *National Diet and Nutrition Survey: adults aged 19 to 64 years. Volume 4: Nutritional status (anthropometry and blood analytes), blood pressure and physical activity.* TSO (London, 2004).

2   The areas included in each of the four analysis 'regions' are given in the response chapter, Chapter 2 of the Technical Report (see Note 9). Definitions of 'regions' are given in the glossary (see Appendix F).

3   Households receiving certain benefits are those where someone in the respondent's household was currently receiving Working Families Tax Credit or had, in the previous 14 days, drawn Income Support or (Income-related) Job Seeker's Allowance. Definitions of 'household' and 'benefits (receiving)' are given in the glossary (see Appendix F).

4   Gregory J, Foster K, Tyler H, Wiseman M. *The Dietary and Nutritional Survey of British Adults.* HMSO (London, 1990).

5   Responsibility for this survey and the National Diet and Nutrition Survey programme transferred from the Ministry of Agriculture, Fisheries and Food to the Food Standards Agency on its establishment in April 2000.

6   Finch S, Doyle W, Lowe C, Bates CJ, Prentice A, Smithers G, Clarke PC. *National Diet and Nutrition Survey: people aged 65 years and over. Volume 1: Report of the diet and nutrition survey.* TSO (London, 1998).

7   Gregory JR, Collins DL, Davies PSW, Hughes JM, Clarke PC. *National Diet and Nutrition Survey: children aged 1½ to 4½ years. Volume 1: Report of the diet and nutrition survey.* HMSO (London, 1995).

8   Gregory JR, Lowe S, Bates CJ, Prentice A, Jackson LV, Smithers G, Wenlock R, Farron M. *National Diet and Nutrition Survey: young people aged 4 to 18 years. Volume 1: Report of the diet and nutrition survey.* TSO (London, 2000).

9   The Technical Report is available online at http:// www.food.gov.uk/science.

10   For further information about the archived data contact:

    The Data Archive
    University of Essex
    Wivenhoe Park
    Colchester
    Essex CO4 3SQ
    UK
    Tel: (UK) 01206 872001
    Fax: (UK) 01206 872003
    Email: archive@essex.ac.uk
    Website: www.data-archive.ac.uk

11   Additional components not reported in this Volume include a seven-day record of bowel movements and self-tooth and amalgam filling count.

12   For more information on the urine analysis, *see* Chapter 4 in Volume 3 (see Note 1(iii)).

13   The potential health risks associated with being overweight vary depending on where the body fat is distributed. Where fat is deposited centrally around the abdominal region rather than around the hip, there is an increased risk of suffering heart disease, diabetes, gallstones, varicose veins and other diseases.

2   Types and quantities of foods consumed

2.1   Introduction

This chapter looks at the types and quantities of foods consumed by respondents in the survey. Most of the information is taken from the seven-day weighed intake dietary records, but some sections are based on information collected in the dietary interview. Differences in consumption of broad food categories are considered by sex, age, region and household receipt of benefits. Data from this survey are also compared to data from the Dietary and Nutritional Survey of British Adults carried out in 1986/87 (1986/87 Adults Survey)[1]. More details about the dietary interview and dietary diary methodology, together with more detailed results from the analysis of food consumption data, are available in Volume 1 of this series[2].

2.2   Foods consumed

Details of how the information recorded in the dietary record was used to derive food consumption figures are provided in Chapter 2 of Volume 1[2], and in Appendix G of the Technical Report[3]. Tables 2.1(a), (b) and (c) show mean amounts consumed during the seven-day recording period, by sex and age, for 26 food categories[4].

Mean intakes are shown based on *all* respondents who kept a dietary record, that is including both *consumers and non-consumers* of each food category, and for *consumers* only. The percentage of diary respondents who consumed items within each food category is also shown (% consumers). For more detailed information on food consumption see Chapter 2 of Volume 1[2].

2.2.1   Types of foods consumed

By sex

Food categories more likely to be consumed by men than by women were:

- fats & oils;
- meat, meat dishes & meat products;
- sugars, preserves & sweet spreads;
- soft drinks, not low calorie; and
- alcoholic drinks.

Food categories less likely to be consumed by men than by women were:

- yogurt & fromage frais;
- fruit (excluding fruit juice); and
- soft drinks, low calorie.

By sex and age

There were also differences in the proportions consuming food categories by age for both men and women. The following highlights differences between the youngest age group, aged 19 to 24 years, and oldest age group, aged 50 to 64 years, only.

- The youngest group of men and women were *more* likely to consume savoury snacks, and soft drinks, not low calorie, and *less* likely to consume eggs & egg dishes, fish & fish dishes and fruit (excluding fruit juice) compared with the oldest group of men and women.
- Men aged 19 to 24 years were *less* likely to have consumed puddings (including dairy desserts & ice-cream) and cheese, and *more* likely to have consumed pasta, rice & other miscellaneous cereals than men aged 50 to 64 years.
- Women aged 19 to 24 years were *less* likely to have consumed breakfast cereals and biscuits, buns, cakes, pastries & fruit pies, and *more* likely to have consumed low calorie soft drinks than those aged 50 to 64 years.

(Tables 2.1(a) to 2.1(c))

2.2.2   Quantities of foods consumed

Table 2.2 lists significant differences by sex and age in the quantity of foods consumed for the categories shown in Tables 2.1(a) to (c)[4]. This table shows differences in the mean amounts consumed for all respondents, that is, including non-consumers.

By sex

Table 2.2 shows that:

- Men consumed larger quantities of many foods compared with women.
- Women consumed larger quantities of fruit (excluding fruit juice) than men.

Table 2.1(a)

Total quantities (grams) of food consumed in seven days by age of respondent: men**

Food category	Men aged (years):								
	19–24			25–34			35–49		
	Mean all	Mean consumers	% consumers	Mean all	Mean consumers	% consumers	Mean all	Mean consumers	% consumers
	g	g	%	g	g	%	g	g	%
Pasta, rice & other miscellaneous cereals***	767	802	96	743	807	92	564	635	89
Bread	727	743	98	862	870	99	883	892	99
Breakfast cereals	108	220	49	230	355	65	205	309	66
Biscuits, buns, cakes, pastries & fruit pies	167	218	77	216	268	81	268	326	82
Puddings (including dairy desserts & ice-cream)	92	301	31	119	291	41	156	277	56
Milk (whole, semi-skimmed, skimmed)	933	1030	91	1541	1605	96	1670	1730	96
Other milk & cream	58	217	27	60	210	28	39	127	31
Cheese	94	150	63	119	151	79	119	148	80
Yogurt & fromage frais	90	309	29	123	419	29	141	423	33
Eggs & egg dishes	129	266	49	153	218	70	145	200	72
Fats & oils	105	112	94	96	102	94	102	109	94
Meat, meat dishes & meat products	1438	1459	99	1462	1482	99	1439	1481	97
Fish & fish dishes	130	280	46	159	260	61	229	312	74
Vegetables & vegetable dishes (excluding potatoes)	665	691	96	854	866	99	1006	1008	100
Potatoes	864	864	100	777	796	98	811	831	98
Savoury snacks	92	146	63	75	112	66	58	101	57
Fruit (excluding fruit juice)	190	410	46	428	633	68	694	834	83
Nuts	1	*	8	22	93	24	20	81	24
Sugars, preserves & sweet spreads	91	112	82	122	162	75	146	200	73
Confectionery	133	202	66	95	141	67	95	145	66
Fruit juice	264	792	33	258	632	41	393	929	42
Soft drinks, not low calorie	2662	2848	94	1336	1701	79	766	1314	58
Soft drinks, low calorie	565	1660	34	837	2113	40	612	1547	40
Alcoholic drinks	3622	4543	80	3994	4878	82	3530	4201	84
Tea, coffee & water[†]	3799	4064	94	6315	6357	100	7440	7463	100
Miscellaneous[††]	322	341	94	367	386	95	379	393	96
Base = number of respondents		108			219			253	

*   Number of consumers is less than 30 & too small to calculate mean values reliably.

**   Data shown in this table may differ from data presented in Tables 2.10(a) and 2.11(a) of Volume 1 due to an error in the application of the dilution factor. Revised Volume 1 tables are available online at www.food.gov.uk.

*** Pasta, rice and other miscellaneous cereals includes pizza.

[†]   Water includes tap water & bottled water, without added sugar or artificial sweeteners. Tea and coffee amounts are as consumed.

[††]   Includes powdered beverages (except tea & coffee), soups, sauces, condiments & artificial sweeteners.

50–64			All men			Food category
Mean all	Mean consumers	% consumers	Mean all	Mean consumers	% consumers	
g	g	%	g	g	%	
397	480	83	587	661	89	Pasta, rice & other miscellaneous cereals***
879	885	99	856	865	99	Bread
280	416	67	222	347	64	Breakfast cereals
332	379	88	261	315	83	Biscuits, buns, cakes, pastries & fruit pies
191	346	55	149	306	49	Puddings (including dairy desserts & ice-cream)
1605	1731	92	1521	1609	94	Milk (whole, semi-skimmed, skimmed)
51	162	32	51	169	30	Other milk & cream
126	152	83	118	150	79	Cheese
154	404	38	134	403	33	Yogurt & fromage frais
185	237	78	157	223	70	Eggs & egg dishes
119	123	96	106	112	95	Fats & oils
1286	1322	97	1398	1430	98	Meat, meat dishes & meat products
297	359	83	218	314	70	Fish & fish dishes
1135	1140	100	961	971	99	Vegetables & vegetable dishes (excluding potatoes)
850	868	98	821	837	98	Potatoes
31	76	40	58	106	55	Savoury snacks
855	987	87	607	806	75	Fruit (excluding fruit juice)
17	82	21	17	81	21	Nuts
152	198	77	134	177	76	Sugars, preserves & sweet spreads
54	114	47	87	144	61	Confectionery
385	798	48	339	795	43	Fruit juice
478	1076	44	1075	1680	64	Soft drinks, not low calorie
388	1500	26	597	1721	35	Soft drinks, low calorie
2983	3917	76	3498	4345	81	Alcoholic drinks
8004	8004	100	6842	6919	99	Tea, coffee & water[†]
470	485	97	396	413	96	Miscellaneous[††]
		253			833	Base = number of respondents

Table 2.1(b)

Total quantities (grams) of food consumed in seven days by age of respondent: women**

Food category	Women aged (years):								
	19–24			25–34			35–49		
	Mean all	Mean consumers	% consumers	Mean all	Mean consumers	% consumers	Mean all	Mean consumers	% consumers
	g	g	%	g	g	%	g	g	%
Pasta, rice & other miscellaneous cereals***	520	584	89	512	560	92	446	530	84
Bread	591	603	98	569	579	99	573	583	98
Breakfast cereals	122	224	55	138	202	69	190	269	71
Biscuits, buns, cakes, pastries & fruit pies	102	156	65	186	222	84	209	242	86
Puddings (including dairy desserts & ice-cream)	123	251	49	112	240	47	131	234	56
Milk (whole, semi-skimmed, skimmed)	1068	1236	87	1137	1196	95	1457	1550	94
Other milk & cream	64	*	28	37	136	27	55	187	29
Cheese	87	132	66	106	133	80	89	122	73
Yogurt & fromage frais	121	387	32	138	326	42	177	400	44
Eggs & egg dishes	92	195	47	88	151	59	113	168	67
Fats & oils	55	64	87	60	64	94	69	76	90
Meat, meat dishes & meat products	946	1030	92	805	925	87	919	990	93
Fish & fish dishes	144	239	61	151	232	65	215	289	74
Vegetables & vegetable dishes (excluding potatoes)	626	639	98	911	924	99	970	980	99
Potatoes	761	788	97	599	618	97	636	656	97
Savoury snacks	83	108	76	64	92	69	41	73	57
Fruit (excluding fruit juice)	379	552	69	521	648	80	687	853	81
Nuts	11	*	17	10	54	19	14	69	19
Sugars, preserves & sweet spreads	52	85	61	75	109	69	87	122	71
Confectionery	89	140	63	77	114	68	80	117	68
Fruit juice	353	701	50	316	625	50	301	690	44
Soft drinks, not low calorie	1705	2179	78	771	1230	63	560	1041	54
Soft drinks, low calorie	1002	1889	53	1185	2054	58	555	1449	38
Alcoholic drinks	1552	2194	71	1069	1554	69	960	1428	67
Tea, coffee & water†	4263	4263	100	6045	6079	100	7468	7535	99
Miscellaneous††	238	252	95	338	357	95	367	388	94
Base = number of respondents			104			210			318

*   *Number of consumers is less than 30 & too small to calculate mean values reliably.*

**   *Data shown in this table may differ from data presented in Tables 2.10(b) and 2.11(b) of Volume 1 due to an error in the application of the dilution factor. Revised Volume 1 tables are available online at www.food.gov.uk.*

*** *Pasta, rice and other miscellaneous cereals includes pizza.*

†   *Water includes tap water & bottled water, without added sugar or artificial sweeteners. Tea and coffee amounts are as consumed.*

††   *Includes powdered beverages (except tea & coffee), soups, sauces, condiments & artificial sweeteners.*

50–64			All women			Food category
Mean all	Mean consumers	% consumers	Mean all	Mean consumers	% consumers	
g	g	%	g	g	%	
317	405	78	433	511	85	Pasta, rice & other miscellaneous cereals***
544	555	98	566	576	98	Bread
245	325	75	186	267	70	Breakfast cereals
254	282	90	204	242	84	Biscuits, buns, cakes, pastries & fruit pies
166	278	59	135	251	54	Puddings (including dairy desserts & ice-cream)
1488	1581	94	1345	1440	93	Milk (whole, semi-skimmed, skimmed)
74	188	39	57	181	32	Other milk & cream
99	125	79	96	127	75	Cheese
209	456	46	171	399	43	Yogurt & fromage frais
135	178	76	111	170	65	Eggs & egg dishes
75	83	91	67	74	91	Fats & oils
832	869	96	870	943	92	Meat, meat dishes & meat products
298	356	83	216	294	73	Fish & fish dishes
1004	1006	100	926	935	99	Vegetables & vegetable dishes (excluding potatoes)
670	695	96	652	674	97	Potatoes
20	51	39	45	80	57	Savoury snacks
1060	1141	93	720	871	83	Fruit (excluding fruit juice)
13	58	23	12	62	20	Nuts
83	122	68	79	115	68	Sugars, preserves & sweet spreads
66	115	57	76	118	64	Confectionery
358	766	47	327	697	47	Fruit juice
416	940	44	702	1254	56	Soft drinks, not low calorie
379	1190	32	705	1650	43	Soft drinks, low calorie
678	1041	65	973	1444	67	Alcoholic drinks
8092	8197	98	6938	6996	99	Tea, coffee & water[†]
389	402	97	351	369	95	Miscellaneous[††]
		259			891	Base = number of respondents

Table 2.1(c)

Total quantities (grams) of food consumed in seven days by age of respondent: all respondents**

Food category	All aged (years):								
	19–24			25–34			35–49		
	Mean all	Mean consumers	% consumers	Mean all	Mean consumers	% consumers	Mean all	Mean consumers	% consumers
	g	g	%	g	g	%	g	g	%
Pasta, rice & other miscellaneous cereals***	646	699	92	630	686	92	498	578	86
Bread	660	674	98	719	728	99	711	721	99
Breakfast cereals	115	222	52	185	278	67	197	286	69
Biscuits, buns, cakes, pastries & fruit pies	135	190	71	201	245	82	235	278	85
Puddings (including dairy desserts & ice-cream)	107	271	40	115	264	44	142	253	56
Milk (whole, semi-skimmed, skimmed)	999	1129	89	1343	1405	96	1551	1631	95
Other milk & cream	61	223	27	48	175	28	48	160	30
Cheese	91	141	65	113	142	80	102	135	76
Yogurt & fromage frais	105	349	30	130	365	36	161	409	39
Eggs & egg dishes	111	232	48	121	188	64	127	183	70
Fats & oils	80	89	90	78	84	94	84	91	92
Meat, meat dishes & meat products	1196	1256	95	1140	1226	93	1149	1213	95
Fish & fish dishes	137	257	53	155	246	86	221	299	74
Vegetables & vegetable dishes (excluding potatoes)	646	665	97	882	894	99	986	993	99
Potatoes	814	827	99	690	709	97	713	734	97
Savoury snacks	87	126	70	69	102	68	49	85	57
Fruit (excluding fruit juice)	283	493	58	473	641	74	690	844	82
Nuts	6	*	12	16	76	21	16	75	22
Sugars, preserves & sweet spreads	72	101	72	99	137	72	113	157	72
Confectionery	111	172	65	86	128	67	86	129	67
Fruit juice	307	738	42	287	628	46	342	794	43
Soft drinks, not low calorie	2193	2550	86	1059	1497	71	651	1168	56
Soft drinks, low calorie	780	1797	43	1007	2079	48	580	1493	39
Alcoholic drinks	2607	3461	75	2562	3395	75	2099	2811	75
Tea, coffee & water†	4027	4165	97	6183	6221	99	7456	7503	99
Miscellaneous††	281	297	94	353	372	95	372	390	95
Base = number of respondents		212			430			570	

*   Number of consumers is less than 30 & too small to calculate mean values reliably.

** Data shown in this table may differ from data presented in Table 2.14 of Volume 1 due to an error in the application of the dilution factor. Revised Volume 1 tables are available online at www.food.gov.uk.

*** Pasta, rice and other miscellaneous cereals includes pizza.

†   Water includes tap water & bottled water, without added sugar or artificial sweeteners. Tea and coffee amounts are as consumed.

††   Includes powdered beverages (except tea & coffee), soups, sauces, condiments & artificial sweeteners.

50–64			All			Food category
Mean all	Mean consumers	% consumers	Mean all	Mean consumers	% consumers	
g	g	%	g	g	%	
356	443	80	507	585	87	Pasta, rice & other miscellaneous cereals***
710	719	99	706	716	99	Bread
263	367	71	203	304	67	Breakfast cereals
293	329	89	231	277	84	Biscuits, buns, cakes, pastries & fruit pies
178	311	57	142	276	51	Puddings (including dairy desserts & ice-cream)
1546	1654	93	1430	1522	94	Milk (whole, semi-skimmed, skimmed)
63	176	36	54	176	31	Other milk & cream
112	138	81	106	138	77	Cheese
182	433	42	153	401	38	Yogurt & fromage frais
160	208	77	133	197	68	Eggs & egg dishes
97	103	94	86	93	93	Fats & oils
1057	1094	96	1125	1186	95	Meat, meat dishes & meat products
297	357	83	217	304	71	Fish & fish dishes
1069	1073	100	943	952	99	Vegetables & vegetable dishes (excluding potatoes)
759	781	97	734	753	97	Potatoes
25	63	39	52	92	56	Savoury snacks
959	1068	90	666	841	79	Fruit (excluding fruit juice)
15	69	22	15	71	20	Nuts
117	162	72	106	147	72	Sugars, preserves & sweet spreads
60	115	52	82	131	62	Confectionery
372	782	47	333	742	45	Fruit juice
446	1007	44	882	1474	60	Soft drinks, not low calorie
384	1327	29	653	1680	39	Soft drinks, low calorie
1818	2574	71	2193	2974	74	Alcoholic drinks
8049	8101	99	6892	6959	99	Tea, coffee & water[†]
429	443	97	373	390	96	Miscellaneous[††]
		512			1724	Base = number of respondents

By sex and age

Table 2.2 also shows significant differences in the amounts consumed by sex and age, comparing the youngest group of men and women, those aged 19 to 24 years, with the oldest group aged 50 to 64 years.

- The youngest group of both men and women consumed larger quantities of pasta, rice & other miscellaneous cereals, savoury snacks and soft drinks, not low calorie, than the oldest age group.
- Men aged 19 to 24 years consumed a significantly larger amount of confectionery, and women in the youngest age group a larger amount of alcoholic drinks, than those aged 50 to 64 years.
- The oldest group of both men and women consumed a larger mean amount of breakfast cereals, biscuits, buns, cakes, pastries & fruit pies, fish & fish dishes, vegetables & vegetable dishes (excluding potatoes), fruit (excluding fruit juice), tea, coffee & water and miscellaneous foods (such as soups, sauces and condiments) than those aged 19 to 24 years.
- Men aged 50 to 64 years consumed a larger mean amount of puddings (including dairy desserts & ice-cream), milk (whole, skimmed, semi-skimmed), nuts and sugars, preserves & sweet spreads than those aged 19 to 24 years.

(Table 2.2)

2.2.3 Variation in the foods eaten by region[5]

Tables D1(a) and D1(b) in Appendix D show the proportions of men and women in each region who consumed different types of food, and the mean amounts consumed, during the seven-day dietary recording period for the 26 food categories[4]. For more detailed information on regional differences in foods consumed, *see* Volume 1, Chapter 2, Section 2.3.5[2].

Overall, there were few consistent differences in the proportions consuming from the different food categories or in the quantities of foods consumed by region. For example, respondents in no one region were more likely to have consumed meat, meat dishes & meat products and less likely to have consumed fruit and vegetables than those in other regions. This may be partly because the numbers of people in each regional group were too low for differences to be statistically significant.

(Tables D1(a) and D1(b), Appendix D)

2.2.4 Variation in the foods eaten by household receipt of benefits[6]

Tables D2(a) and D2(b) in Appendix D show the proportions of men and women consuming different types of food, and the mean amounts consumed, during the seven-day dietary recording period according to whether the respondent's household was in receipt of certain state benefits (benefit households). For more detailed information on differences in foods consumed by household receipt of benefits *see* Volume 1, Chapter 2, Section 2.3.6[2].

- Both men and women living in benefit households were less likely to have consumed a number of foods compared to those living in non-benefit households. These include:
  - puddings (including dairy desserts & ice cream);
  - yogurt & fromage frais;
  - fruit (excluding fruit juice); and
  - alcoholic drinks.
- Men in benefit households were less likely to have consumed:
  - nuts; and
  - fruit juice.
- Women in benefit households were less likely to have consumed:
  - breakfast cereals;
  - biscuits, buns, cakes, pastries & fruit pies;
  - other milk & cream;
  - cheese; and
  - fish & fish dishes.

(Tables D2(a) and D2(b), Appendix D)

Table 2.2

Main differences in the total quantity of foods consumed by men and women, including non-consumers

Greater quantity eaten by:

All men (compared with all women)	All women (compared with all men)
Pasta, rice & other miscellaneous cereals*	Fruit (excluding fruit juice)
Bread	
Biscuits, buns, cakes, pastries & fruit pies	
Milk (whole, semi-skimmed, skimmed)	
Cheese	
Eggs & egg dishes	
Fats & oils	
Meat, meat dishes & meat products	
Potatoes	
Savoury snacks	
Sugars, preserves & sweet spreads	
Soft drinks, not low calorie	
Alcoholic drinks	

Greater quantity eaten by:

Men aged 19 to 24 years (compared with men 50 to 64 years)	Men aged 50 to 64 years (compared with men 19 to 24 years)
Pasta, rice & other miscellaneous cereals*	Breakfast cereals
Savoury snacks	Biscuits, buns, cakes, pastries & fruit pies
Soft drinks, not low calorie	Puddings (including dairy desserts & ice cream)
Confectionery	Milk (whole, semi-skimmed, skimmed)
	Fish & fish dishes
	Vegetables & vegetable dishes (excluding potatoes)
	Fruit (excluding fruit juice)
	Nuts
	Sugars, preserves & sweet spreads
	Tea, coffee & water**
	Miscellaneous food items***

Greater quantity eaten by:

Women aged 19 to 24 years (compared with women 50 to 64 years)	Women aged 50 to 64 years (compared with women 19 to 24 years)
Pasta, rice & other miscellaneous cereals*	Breakfast cereals
Savoury snacks	Biscuits, buns, cakes, pastries & fruit pies
Soft drinks, not low calorie	Fish & fish dishes
Alcoholic drinks	Vegetables & vegetable dishes (excluding potatoes)
	Fruit (excluding fruit juice)
	Tea, coffee & water**
	Miscellaneous food items***

*   *Pasta, rice & other miscellaneous cereals includes pizza.*
**   *Water includes tap water & bottled water, without added sugar or artificial sweeteners. Tea and coffee are as consumed.*
***   *Includes powdered beverages (except tea & coffee), soups, sauces, condiments & artificial sweeteners.*

2.3 Fruit and vegetables consumed

2.3.1 Background

A key feature of the Government's framework for reducing early deaths from coronary heart disease and cancer and reducing health inequalities among the general population is to improve access to and increase the consumption of fruit and vegetables. The World Health Organization and the UK's Committee on Medical Aspects of Food and Nutrition policy recommend eating at least five portions (400g) of fruit and vegetables a day. This recommendation forms the basis of the five-a-day programme, part of the action intended to achieve these targets[7].

The five-a-day message is to eat at least 5 portions of a variety of fruit and vegetables each day. Fresh, frozen, chilled, canned, 100% juice and dried fruit all count. However a glass of fruit juice, and a portion of beans or pulses (such as chickpeas or lentils), each count as one portion only, regardless of how much is actually consumed per day[8]. Potatoes, yams and cassavas do not count, as they are 'starchy foods'.

In *practical* terms a portion of fruit or vegetables is, for example:

- a medium sized apple, banana or similar sized fruit
- two small satsumas or similar sized fruit
- half a grapefruit or avocado
- a slice of large fruit such as melon or pineapple
- 1 cupful of grapes, cherries or berries
- three heaped tablespoons of vegetables
- three heaped tablespoons of beans or other pulses
- one glass of fruit juice
- a dessert bowl of salad.

Fruit and vegetable consumption in this survey has been examined using the definition of fruit and vegetables used within the five-a-day programme. Five portions or 400g of fruit and vegetables per day equates to 80g per portion, and this is the definition of portion size used when analysing the data. Fruit and vegetable consumption in the following section is defined as:

- daily consumption of fruit and vegetables, including those in selected composite dishes[9], and including all fruit juice consumed as one portion only, and similarly all baked beans and other pulses consumed as one portion only[8].

More details on the calculation of fruit and vegetable intake and what fruit and vegetables are included, and excluded, can be found in Volume 1[2].

2.3.2 Portions of fruit and vegetables consumed by sex and age of respondent

Table 2.3 shows the average number of portions of fruit and vegetables consumed per day for all respondents including non-consumers. Figure 2.1 shows the mean number of portions of fruit and vegetables consumed per day by sex and age compared with the recommendation of at least five portions per day.

- Men and women consumed, on average, fewer than three portions of fruit and vegetables a day, well below the five-a-day recommended (2.7 for men and 2.9 for women).
- 13% of men and 15% of women met the five-a-day recommendation, consuming five or more portions of fruit and vegetables a day.
- Men and women aged 19 to 24 years consumed fewer portions of fruit and vegetables than those aged 50 to 64 years. Men and women in the youngest group consumed, on average, 1.3 and 1.8 portions of fruit and vegetables per day respectively, compared with 3.6 and 3.8 portions for men and women in the oldest group.
- None of the men, and 4% of the women, in the youngest group met the five-a-day recommendation, compared with 24% of men and 22% of women in the oldest group.
- 21% of men and 15% of women, overall, consumed no fruit during the survey period. This proportion was higher for the youngest group of men and women, 45% and 27% respectively (data not shown, *see* Volume 1, Chapter 2, Section 2.4.5[2]).

(Table 2.3, Figure 2.1)

Table 2.3

Proportion of respondents consuming portions* of fruit and vegetables, including composite dishes**, by sex and age of respondent

Average daily number of portions of fruit and vegetables and one portion fruit juice and/or baked beans or other pulses, including composite dishes**, consumed	Men aged (years):				All men	Women aged (years):				All women	All
	19–24	25–34	35–49	50–64		19–24	25–34	35–49	50–64		
	cum %	cum %	cum %	cum %	cum %	cum %	cum %	cum %	cum %	cum %	cum %
None	6	1	0	1	1	2	1	1	0	1	1
Less than one portion	38	27	14	7	18	36	19	16	7	16	17
Less than two portions	86	54	36	29	45	64	46	41	20	39	42
Less than three portions	95	76	59	45	64	83	71	61	44	61	62
Less than four portions	95	86	75	60	76	96	82	73	60	74	75
Less than five portions	100	93	86	76	87	96	91	83	78	85	86
All		100	100	100	100	100	100	100	100	100	100
Base	108	219	253	253	833	104	210	318	259	891	1724
Mean number of portions consumed (average value)	1.3	2.2	3.0	3.6	2.7	1.8	2.4	2.9	3.8	2.9	2.8
Median number of portions consumed	1.3	1.8	2.6	3.4	2.2	1.6	2.1	2.4	3.3	2.4	2.3
Standard deviation	1.03	1.61	1.87	2.21	1.99	1.33	1.71	1.98	2.20	2.02	2.01

*   Portions include fruit and vegetables (80g per portion) and one portion fruit juice and/or baked beans or other pulses.

** Composite dishes were for fruit: fruit pies, and for vegetables: vegetable dishes, including for example vegetable lasagne, cauliflower cheese and vegetable samosas.

Figure 2.1

Mean number of portions* of fruit and vegetables consumed daily compared with five-a-day recommendation by sex and age of respondent

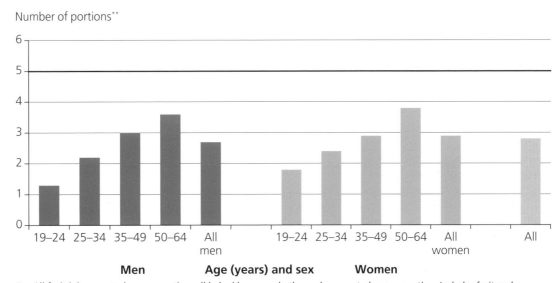

*   All fruit juice counted as one portion; all baked beans and other pulses counted as one portion. Includes fruit and vegetables in selected composite dishes.

** It is recommended that at least five portions of fruit and vegetables are consumed daily.

2.3.3 Portions of fruit and vegetables consumed by region[5]

There were no significant regional differences for men or women in the mean number of portions of fruit and vegetables consumed, in the proportion who consumed five or more portions of fruit and vegetables per day, or in the proportion who had eaten no fruit and vegetables (data not shown; *see* Volume 1[2]).

2.3.4 Portions of fruit and vegetables consumed by household receipt of benefits[6]

Figure 2.2 shows the mean number of portions of fruit and vegetables consumed per day by sex and whether someone in the respondent's household was receiving certain state benefits.

- On average, men and women in benefit households consumed fewer portions of fruit and vegetables per day (2.1 and 1.9 respectively) than those in non-benefit households (2.8 and 3.1 respectively).
- A lower proportion of women in benefit households met the five-a-day recommendation, 4%, compared with 17% of women in non-benefit households (data not shown, *see* Volume 1[2]).

(Figure 2.2)

2.4 Dietary interview data

During the dietary interview respondents were asked if they were taking any dietary supplements, for example, vitamin tablets[10]. They were also asked if they were on a diet to lose weight and whether they were vegetarian or vegan. Table 2.4 shows the breakdown of responses to these questions.

Dietary Supplements

- 35% of respondents reported taking dietary supplements.
- Women were more likely than men to report taking supplements (40% of women overall, rising to over half, 55%, of the oldest group of women).
- The most popular dietary supplements taken were cod liver oil and other fish-based supplements, and multivitamins and multiminerals (*see* Volume 1, Chapter 2, Table 2.6).

Dieting

- 17% of respondents reported being on a diet to lose weight.
- Women were more likely than men to report being on a diet (24% of women compared with 10% of men).

Figure 2.2

Mean number of portions of fruit and vegetables consumed daily compared with five-a-day recommendation by household receipt of benefits and sex of respondent[*]

Number of portions[**]

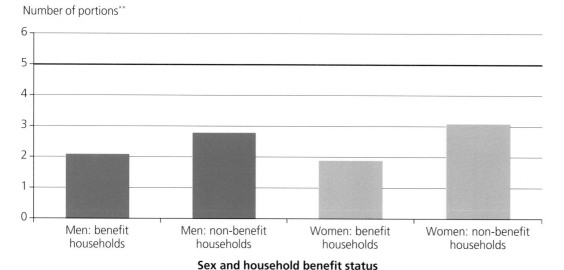

Sex and household benefit status

* All fruit juice counted as one portion; all baked beans and other pulses counted as one portion. Includes fruit and vegetables in selected composite dishes.
** It is recommended that at least five portions of fruit and vegetables are consumed daily.

- There were no age differences for men or women in the proportions who reported dieting to lose weight.

Vegetarian/Vegan

- One in twenty respondents, 5%, reported being vegetarian or vegan.
- Women were more likely than men to report being vegetarian/vegan (7% of women overall compared with 2% of men).
- About 11% of younger women aged 19 to 34 years reported being vegetarian or vegan.

Respondents who reported being vegetarian or vegan were asked what foods they avoided (data not shown):

- all said they avoided red meat;
- 92% avoided white meat;
- 48% said they did not eat fish;
- 29% said they avoided all animal products; and
- 21% said they avoided eating eggs.

(Table 2.4)

2.5 Comparison with 1986/87 Adults Survey

Tables D3(a), (b) and (c) in Appendix D show food consumption figures for this current NDNS compared with figures from the 1986/87 Adults Survey[1]. Comparisons are made between comparable age groups in the two surveys. It should be noted that in the 1986/87 Adults Survey the youngest age group was adults aged 16 to 24 years, while in the current NDNS the youngest age group is adults aged 19 to 24 years. This should be borne in mind where there are differences between these groups. A summary of the methodology and findings from the 1986/87 Adults Survey is given in Appendix S of the Technical Report[3].

Data are presented for comparable food groups[11]. Mean intakes are shown based on *all* respondents who kept a dietary record, that is including both *consumers and non-consumers* of each food group, and for *consumers* only. The percentage of diary respondents who consumed items within each food group during the dietary recording period is also shown (% consumers).

(Tables D3(a) to D3(c), Appendix D)

Table 2.4

Percentage of respondents who reported (a) currently taking dietary supplements (including fluoride), (b) dieting to lose weight, (c) being vegetarian or vegan, by sex and age of respondent

Responding sample   *Percentages*

	Percentage taking supplements	Percentage reporting dieting to lose weight	Percentage reporting being vegetarian or vegan	Base
Sex and age of respondent				
Men aged (years):				
19–24	22	9	3	142
25–34	28	6	1	287
35–49	29	12	3	330
50–64	34	13	2	330
All men	29	10	2	1088
Women aged (years):				
19–24	31	21	12	136
25–34	34	28	11	275
35–49	36	25	5	415
50–64	55	20	4	337
All women	40	24	7	1163
All	35	17	5	2251

2.5.1 Types of foods consumed

Table 2.5 summarises significant differences between the 1986/87 Adults Survey and this survey in the proportions consuming different food items. Overall, a large number of foods were more likely to have been consumed by respondents in the 1986/87 Adults Survey compared with respondents in the current NDNS.

Food categories more likely to have been consumed by respondents in the 1986/87 Adults Survey (compared with the current NDNS):

- biscuits, buns, cakes, pastries & fruit pies;
- puddings (including dairy desserts & ice-creams);
- milk;
- cheese;
- eggs & egg dishes;
- fats & oils;
- meat, meat dishes & meat products;
- fish & fish dishes;
- sugars, preserves & sweet spreads; and
- tea & water.

Food categories more likely to have been consumed by respondents in the 2000/01 NDNS (compared with the 1986/87 Adults Survey):

- pasta, rice & other miscellaneous cereals;
- breakfast cereals;
- yogurt & fromage frais;
- savoury snacks;
- nuts;
- soft drinks, low calorie; and
- alcoholic drinks.

Table 2.5 also shows that, within these broad food categories, respondents in the 1986/87 Adults Survey were more likely to eat a range of foods compared with respondents in the current survey. These include:

- wholemeal bread;
- ice cream;
- whole milk;
- butter;
- a wide range of meat, meat dishes & meat products;
- a range of vegetables;
- table sugar; and
- fortified wine.

There were fewer foods which were more likely to be eaten by adults in the current survey compared with adults in the 1986/87 Adults Survey. Those that were include:

- pasta;
- rice;
- white bread;
- semi-skimmed milk;
- chicken and turkey;
- oily fish;
- shellfish;
- salad vegetables;
- bananas; and
- wine.

By sex and age

Tables D4(a) and D4(b) in Appendix D summarise significant differences by sex and age in the proportions consuming different foods between the two surveys. Overall, many of the differences in food consumption patterns between the two surveys described above are also evident when comparisons are made by sex and age.

(Table 2.5)
(Tables D4(a) and D4(b), Appendix D)

2.5.2 Quantities of foods consumed

Tables D5, D6(a) and D6(b) in Appendix D summarise significant differences in quantities of foods consumed between the two surveys, by sex and age. These differences have been calculated on mean amounts consumed for all respondents, that is, including non-consumers.

Significant differences in the mean amounts consumed between the two surveys show a similar pattern to that seen above for types of foods consumed.

Several factors will have contributed to differences in the types and quantities of foods consumed between the two surveys. For example, there has been an increase in the types of foods available, for example, pasta and coated chicken and turkey products, and an increase in eating out.

(Tables D5, D6(a) and D6(b), Appendix D)

2.5.3 Supplements

Respondents were asked at the dietary interview if they were taking any extra vitamins, minerals, or other dietary supplements (*see* Volume 1, Chapter 2, Section 2.2.4[2])[10]. In the 2000/01 survey, 40% of women and 29% of men reported taking supplements. In the 1986/87 Adults Survey 17% of women and 9% of men reported taking supplements. Women were more likely to report taking dietary supplements than men in both surveys and supplement taking was most common in the oldest group of women in both the 1986/87 Adults Survey and the current survey, 23% and 55% respectively.

Table 2.5

Main differences in the eating behaviour of respondents in 1986/87 Adults Survey* and those in the 2000/01 NDNS: all respondents

Foods more likely to be eaten by respondents in:

1986/87 Adults Survey (compared with 2000/01 NDNS)		2000/01 NDNS (compared with 1986/87 Adults Survey)	
Food category	Food type	Food category	Food type
	Wholemeal bread	Pasta, rice & other miscellaneous cereals**	Pasta
			Rice
Biscuits, buns, cakes, pastries & fruit pies	Biscuits		White bread
	Fruit pies		
	Buns, cakes & pastries	Breakfast cereals	
			Semi-skimmed milk
Puddings (including dairy desserts & ice cream)	Ice cream		
		Yogurt & fromage frais	
Milk***	Whole milk		Coated chicken & turkey
			Chicken & turkey dishes
Cheese			
			Oily fish****
Eggs & egg dishes			Shellfish
Fats & oils	Butter		Other raw & salad vegetables
			Tomatoes - not raw
Meat & meat products	Bacon & ham		
	Beef, veal & dishes		Potato products, not fried
	Lamb & dishes		
	Pork & dishes	Savoury snacks	
	Liver, liver products & dishes		Bananas
	Sausages	Nuts	
	Meat pies & pastries		
	Other meat & meat products	Soft drinks, low calorie†	
Fish & fish dishes	White fish	Alcoholic drinks††	Wine††
	Peas		
	Leafy green vegetables		
	Carrots - not raw		
	Other vegetables		
	Fried/roast potatoes & fried potato products		
	Other potatoes & potato dishes		
	Canned fruit in syrup		
Sugars, preserves & sweet spreads	Table sugar		
	Preserves		
	Fortified wine		
	Cider & perry††		
Tea & water†††			

* Gregory JR et al. The Dietary and Nutritional Survey of British Adults. HMSO (London, 1990).
** Pasta, rice & other miscellaneous cereals includes pizza.
*** Includes whole milk, semi-skimmed milk and skimmed milk only. Other milks and creams are excluded as data are not comparable between the two surveys due to differences in the dietary recording methodology.
**** Oily fish includes canned tuna.
† Figures for soft drinks, low calorie and not low calorie, are as consumed, that is includes concentrated drinks plus diluent.
†† Includes low-alcohol variations.
††† Water includes tap water, and bottled water without added sugar or artificial sweeteners. Coffee is excluded as data are not comparable due to differences in the dietary recording methodology.

2.6 Summary

Foods consumed

There were many differences in types and quantities of foods consumed by sex and age. For example:

- Men were more likely than women to have consumed meat, meat dishes & meat products and women more likely than men to have consumed fruit (excluding fruit juice).
- The youngest group of men and women were more likely to have consumed savoury snacks and soft drinks, not low calorie, whereas those in the oldest age group were more likely to have consumed fish & fish dishes and fruit (excluding fruit juice).
- There are few consistent differences in patterns of consumption by region.
- Men and women in benefit households were less likely to consume a number of foods compared with those in non-benefit households, including, for example, fruit (excluding fruit juice) and alcoholic drinks.

Fruit & vegetables

- On average, men consumed 2.7 portions of fruit and vegetables per day, and women 2.9 portions.
- The youngest group of men and women consumed fewer portions of fruit and vegetables than those in the oldest group.
- Overall, 13% of men and 15% of women met the five-a-day recommendation.
- 21% of men and 15% of women consumed no fruit during the survey period.
- Men and women in benefit households consumed fewer portions of fruit and vegetables (2.1 and 1.9 respectively) than those in non-benefit households (2.8 and 3.1 respectively).

Dietary supplements

- 35% of respondents reported taking dietary supplements, with women more likely to report this than men. The most common supplements were: cod liver oil & other fish-based supplements, multivitamins and multiminerals.

Dieting

- 17% of respondents reported being on a diet to lose weight, with women more likely to report this than men.

Comparison with the 1986/87 Adults Survey

- Overall, a large number of foods were more likely to be consumed in the 1986/87 Adults Survey than in the 2000/01 NDNS, including, biscuits, buns, cakes, pastries & fruit pies, meat & meat products and fish & fish dishes.
- Respondents in the present survey were more likely to have consumed, for example, breakfast cereals, savoury snacks, soft drinks (low calorie) and alcoholic drinks.

References and endnotes

1. Gregory J, Foster K, Tyler H, Wiseman M. *The Dietary and Nutritional Survey of British Adults.* HMSO (London, 1990).

2. Henderson L, Gregory J, Swan G. *National Diet and Nutrition Survey: adults aged 19 to 64 years. Volume 1: Types and quantities of foods consumed.* TSO (London, 2002).

3. The Technical Report is available online at http://www.food.gov.uk/science.

4. Volume 1 presents food consumption data for 107 individual food groups. For this summary volume, food consumption data have been amalgamated into 26 broader categories, as shown in Tables 2.1(a), 2.1(b), 2.1(c), 2.2 and Tables D1(a) to D2(b) in Appendix D.

5. The areas included in each of the four analysis 'regions' are given in the response chapter, Chapter 2 of the Technical Report (*see* Note 3). Definitions of 'regions' are given in the glossary (*see* Appendix F).

6. Households receiving certain benefits are those where someone in the respondent's household was currently receiving Working Families Tax Credit or had, in the previous 14 days, drawn Income Support or (Income-related) Job Seeker's Allowance. Definitions of 'household' and 'benefits (receiving)' are given in the glossary (*see* Appendix F).

7. The five-a-day programme is being developed by the Department of Health, in conjunction with the Food Standards Agency, the Department for Environment, Food and Rural Affairs (DEFRA), the Department for Education and Skills (DfES), and the Health Development Agency. Consumer, health, education and parent organisations are also involved along with the food industry. More information can be obtained at http://www.dh.gov.uk/PolicyAndGuidance/HealthAndSocialCareTopics/FiveADay.

8. Juice (fruit or vegetable) only counts as 1 portion a day, regardless of how much is drunk, because it has very little fibre. Also, the juicing process 'squashes' the natural sugars out of the cells that normally contain them, and this means that drinking juice in between meals isn't good for teeth. Pulses contain fibre, but they don't give the same mixture of vitamins, minerals and

other nutrients as fruit and vegetables. So in order to get a healthy balance, it is important to ensure a variety of fruit and vegetables is consumed (*see* www.dh.gov.uk/ PolicyAndGuidance/HealthAndSocialCareTopics/ FiveADay).

9   Composite dishes included in the analysis of fruit and vegetable consumption were for fruit: fruit pies, and for vegetables: vegetable dishes, including vegetable lasagne, cauliflower cheese and vegetable samosas. Further details are given in Volume 1, Appendix A 'Fruit and vegetables' (*see* Note 2).

10   Respondents were asked at the dietary interview if they were taking any extra vitamins, minerals, including fluoride, or other dietary supplements or herbal preparations, including prescribed or non-prescribed supplements. Those who reported taking supplements were asked to give a description of the product, including the brand name and strength, form, dose and frequency.

11   Food consumption data from the 1986/87 Adults Survey has been re-calculated, and the data for both surveys re-structured into specific food groups to allow comparisons

3 Nutrient intakes

3.1 Introduction

In this chapter, data are presented on the intakes of selected nutrients by those respondents in the survey who kept a dietary record for the full seven days. Intakes are presented for energy, protein, total carbohydrate, non-milk extrinsic sugars, non-starch polysaccharides (that is, fibre), total fat, saturated fatty acids and a key selection of vitamins and minerals.

The information from the dietary record was linked to a nutrient databank and nutrient intakes were calculated from the quantities of foods consumed. Nutrient intakes across the seven-day dietary recording period have been used to produce an average daily intake for each nutrient. Intakes of vitamins and minerals presented in this volume exclude any contribution from supplements. However, the effect of dietary supplements on intakes of vitamins and minerals is also discussed. No attempt has been made to adjust the nutrient intakes presented here to take account of under-reporting[1]. Nutrient intakes from this survey are also compared with intakes as recorded in the Dietary and Nutritional Survey of British Adults aged 16 to 64 years carried out in 1986/87 (1986/87 Adults Survey)[2].

Having a low intake of a nutrient during the survey week does not necessarily mean that an individual is deficient in that nutrient. An individual's status can be confirmed for some nutrients by analysis of a blood sample for biochemical indices of the levels of the nutrient available in the body (*see* Chapter 4 for results from the analysis of respondents' blood samples).

More detailed information on intakes of nutrients and food sources of nutrients, including those not discussed in this volume[3], can be found in Volumes 2 and 3[4,5].

3.1.1 Dietary Reference Values (DRVs)

Dietary Reference Values (DRVs) were defined by the Department of Health in the report *Dietary Reference Values for Food Energy and Nutrients for the United Kingdom*, published in 1991[6]. These include Estimated Average Requirements (EARs), Reference Nutrient Intake values (RNI) and Lower Reference Nutrient Intake values (LRNI).

Estimates of energy requirements for different populations are termed 'Estimated Average Requirements' (EARs) and are defined as the energy intake estimated to meet the *average* requirements of the population group. EARs were set by the Committee on Medical Aspects of Food Policy (COMA) and were based largely on energy expenditure data. EARs for energy are shown in Table 3.1. DRVs for carbohydrates and fats, based on population average intakes as a percentage of energy intake, are shown in Table 3.2. For fat, saturated fatty acids and non-milk extrinsic sugars, these are maximum guidelines based on population average intakes as a percentage of energy intake. For example, average total fat intake should contribute no more than 35% of food energy intake for the population. For total carbohydrate, 50% of food energy should come from carbohydrate as a population average.

Reference Nutrient Intake values (RNIs) have been published for protein. RNIs and Lower Reference Nutrient Intake values (LRNIs) have been published for a range of vitamins and minerals. The RNI for a nutrient is an amount of that nutrient that is sufficient, or more than sufficient, for about 97% of the people in that group. If the average intake of the group is at the RNI, then the risk of deficiency in the group is judged to be very small. However, if the average intake is lower than the RNI then it is possible that some of the group will have an intake below their requirement. This is even more likely if a proportion of the group have an intake below the LRNI. The LRNI for a vitamin or mineral is the amount of that nutrient that is enough for only the few people in a group who have low needs. For further definitions of the RNI and LRNI *see* Department of Health (1991)[6,7]. The RNI for protein is shown in Table 3.2 and the relevant RNIs and LRNIs for the vitamins and minerals discussed in this chapter are shown in Table 3.3.

(Tables 3.1 to 3.3)

3.2 Energy and macronutrients (protein, total carbohydrate, non-milk extrinsic sugars, non-starch polysaccharides, total fat and saturated fatty acids)

This section looks at mean daily intakes of energy and macronutrients, that is protein, total carbohydrate, non-milk extrinsic sugars, non-starch polysaccharides, total fat and saturated fatty acids for respondents in this survey, and how they compare to DRVs, by sex and age. Data are presented on the foods that are major contributors to intakes of these nutrients. A brief explanation of the different macronutrients is given first.

Table 3.1

Estimated Average Requirements (EARs) for Energy*

Age (years)	EARs (MJ/d) (kcal/d)	
	Men	Women
19–50	10.60 (2,550)	8.10 (1,940)
51–59	10.60 (2,550)	8.00 (1,900)
60–64	9.93 (2,380)	7.99 (1,900)

* Source: Department of Health. Report on Health and Social Subjects: 41. Dietary Reference Values for Food Energy and Nutrients for the United Kingdom. HMSO (London, 1991).

Table 3.2

Dietary Reference Values for protein, carbohydrate (including non-starch polysaccharides) and fat for adults*

Nutrient	
Protein (RNI g/day)	
Men 19 to 50 years	55.5
Men over 50 years	53.3
Women 19 to 50 years	45.0
Women over 50 years	46.5
Non-starch polysaccharide (g/day)	18
Intakes as % of total energy (% food energy)	
Total carbohydrate	47 (50)
Non-milk extrinsic sugars	10 (11)
Total fat	33 (35)
Saturated fatty acids	10 (11)

* Source: Department of Health. Report on Health and Social Subjects: 41. Dietary Reference Values for Food Energy and Nutrients for the United Kingdom. HMSO (London, 1991).

Table 3.3

Reference Nutrient Intakes (RNIs) and Lower Reference Nutrient Intakes (LRNIs) for vitamins and minerals*

Vitamins & minerals	Units	RNI and LRNI by sex and age (years)**							
		Men				Women			
		19 to 50		51 to 64		19 to 50		51 to 64	
		RNI	LRNI	RNI	LRNI	RNI	LRNI	RNI	LRNI
Vitamins									
Vitamin A (retinol equivalents)	µg/d	700	300	700	300	600	250	600	250
Thiamin***	mg/d	1.0	0.6	0.9	0.5	0.8	0.4	0.8	0.4
Riboflavin	mg/d	1.3	0.8	1.3	0.8	1.1	0.8	1.1	0.8
Niacin***	mg/d	17	11	16	10	13	9	12	8
Vitamin B_6****	mg/d	1.4	1.0	1.4	1.0	1.2	0.8	1.2	0.8
Vitamin B_{12}	µg/d	1.5	1.0	1.5	1.0	1.5	1.0	1.5	1.0
Folate	µg/d	200	100	200	100	200	100	200	100
Vitamin C	mg/d	40	10	40	10	40	10	40	10
Minerals									
Total iron	mg/d	8.7	4.7	8.7	4.7	14.8	8.0	8.7	4.7
Calcium	mg/d	700	400	700	400	700	400	700	400
Magnesium	mg/d	300	190	300	190	270	150	270	150
Potassium	mg/d	3500	2000	3500	2000	3500	2000	3500	2000
Zinc	mg/d	9.5	5.5	9.5	5.5	7.0	4.0	7.0	4.0
Iodine	µg/d	140	70	140	70	140	70	140	70
Copper	mg/d	1.2	n/a	1.2	n/a	1.2	n/a	1.2	n/a

*   Source: Department of Health. Report on Health and Social Subjects: 41. Dietary Reference Values for Food Energy and Nutrients for the United Kingdom. HMSO (London, 1991).
**   The age groups presented represent those for which different RNI and LRNI values are calculated.
*** Calculated values based on Estimated Average Requirements (EARs) for energy; calculated values from quoted LRNIs mg/1000kcal.
**** Based on protein providing 14.7% of the EAR for energy. Calculated values from quoted LRNIs µg/g protein.
n/a no reference value set.

3.2.1 Introduction

Energy

Energy is required for the body to function and be active. Energy is derived from the intake of carbohydrate, fat, protein and alcohol in the diet. Total energy includes energy derived from alcohol, food energy excludes energy derived from alcohol.

Protein

Protein is a vital component of all cells in the body and is needed in the diet for growth and repair of the body. Excess protein can be used to provide energy.

Carbohydrate

There are three major groups of carbohydrates in foods – sugars, starches and non-starch polysaccharides. Sugars and starches are major contributors to energy intakes. For the purposes of this survey, total carbohydrate consists of non-milk extrinsic sugars, intrinsic and milk sugars and starch (non-starch polysaccharides are classified separately). Intrinsic sugars are those sugars that are located within the cell structure of a food, e.g. fresh, unprocessed fruit. Milk sugars are those that are occur naturally in milk and milk products. Intrinsic and milk sugars (not discussed in this summary volume) are not thought to be harmful to teeth. Non-milk extrinsic sugars are not contained within the cell structure of a food, either because they have been added to a food in the form of, for example, table sugar or honey, or because the food has been processed which has released (otherwise intrinsic) sugars from the cell structure, for example, fruit juice. Non-milk extrinsic sugars are those sugars that are believed to be harmful to teeth.

Non-starch polysaccharides

Non-starch polysaccharides fall under the more familiar term 'dietary fibre'. They are important in helping to maintain bowel health and prevent constipation. The type of non-starch polysaccharide found in fruit, vegetables, oats and pulses, for example, has also been shown to help lower blood cholesterol levels.

Fat and fatty acids

Fats are important in the diet as they provide energy and essential nutrients, including some vitamins, and improve the palatability of foods. There are two main types of fat, saturated and unsaturated fats. Unsaturated fats can be further divided into monounsaturated fats,

polyunsaturated fats and *trans* unsaturated fats. Saturated fats are found in products of animal origin, principally dairy and meat products, and are often called 'bad fats'. This is because they can increase blood cholesterol levels and the risk of coronary heart disease. Monounsaturated fats and polyunsaturated fats are often called 'good fats', because replacing saturated fats with these fats can help to lower blood cholesterol levels and also because polyunsaturated fats provide fats which are essential to life. This volume focuses on total fat and saturated fatty acids only. Further details on other fatty acids can be found in Volume 2[4].

3.2.2 Intakes of energy and macronutrients

Table 3.4 shows mean intakes of total energy, protein, total carbohydrate, non-milk extrinsic sugars, non-starch polysaccharides, total fat and saturated fatty acids by sex and age and how they compare to DRVs.

- Men have higher intakes of total energy and most macronutrients than women.
- There were no age differences in total energy intake for men or women, and few differences in intakes of macronutrients by age.

Comparing intakes of these macronutrients with the relevant DRV allows us to look at the adequacy of these macronutrient intakes for, and between, each sex/age group (*see* Table 3.4; Figures 3.1, 3.2 and 3.3).

- Mean daily **total energy** intakes were below EARs for each sex and age group.
- Average **protein** intakes for all sex and age groups were above the RNI.
- The mean percentage of food energy derived from **total carbohydrate** was near the DRV for all sex and age groups.
- The mean percentage of food energy derived from **non-milk extrinsic sugars** was above the DRV for all sex and age groups except for the oldest group of women, and was highest in the youngest group of men and women (*see* Figure 3.1).
- Mean daily intake of **non-starch polysaccharides** was below the recommended average intake of 18g per day for all sex and age groups. A higher proportion of women than men had intakes of non-starch polysaccharides less than 18g/day. Men and women aged 19 to 34 years were more likely to have a mean daily intake of non-starch polysaccharides below 18g than those in the oldest age group. In addition, men aged 19 to 24 years were more likely to have intakes less than

Table 3.4

Average daily intake of energy and macronutrients and intakes compared with Dietary Reference Values (DRVs) by sex and age of respondent*

Energy and macronutrients	Men aged (years):				All men	Women aged (years):				All women
	19–24	25–34	35–49	50–64		19–24	25–34	35–49	50–64	
Total energy intake (MJ)										
Mean (average value)	9.44	9.82	9.93	9.55	9.72	7.00	6.61	6.96	6.91	6.87
% of Estimated Average Requirements**	89%	93%	94%	92%	92%	86%	82%	86%	87%	85%
Protein										
Mean (average value)	77.8	90.6	90.1	88.8	88.2	59.9	58.7	65.1	67.4	63.7
% of RNI	140%	163%	162%	166%	161%	133%	131%	145%	145%	140%
Total carbohydrate*										
Mean (average value)	273	277	279	269	275	206	196	206	203	203
% of food energy	49.0%	47.7%	47.5%	47.4%	47.7%	49.1%	48.7%	48.6%	48.1%	48.5%
Non-milk extrinsic sugars[†]										
Mean (average value)	96	80	78	70	79	60	49	51	48	51
% of food energy	17.4%	13.9%	13.1%	12.2%	13.6%	14.2%	11.8%	11.8%	11.0%	11.9%
Non-starch polysaccharides										
Mean (average value)	12.3	14.6	15.7	16.4	15.2	10.6	11.6	12.8	14.0	12.6
% with intakes < 18g	94%	77%	70%	61%	72%	96%	92%	85%	80%	87%
Total fat[††]										
Mean (average value)	85.8	87.1	88.3	84.5	86.5	63.9	59.8	61.9	61.2	61.4
% of food energy	36.0%	35.8%	35.9%	35.6%	35.8%	35.5%	35.4%	34.7%	34.5%	34.9%
Saturated fatty acids[††]										
Mean (average value)	32.3	32.2	33.4	32.0	32.5	23.5	22.4	23.6	23.7	23.3
% of food energy	13.5%	13.2%	13.5%	13.4%	13.4%	12.9%	13.2%	13.2%	13.3%	13.2%
Base	*108*	*219*	*253*	*253*	*833*	*104*	*210*	*318*	*259*	*891*

* Source: Department of Health. Report on Health and Social Subjects: 41. Dietary Reference Values for Food Energy and Nutrients for the United Kingdom. HMSO (London, 1991).

** Energy intake as a percentage of EAR was calculated for each respondent using the EAR appropriate for sex and age.

*** The Dietary Reference Value for total carbohydrate is that the population average intake should contribute 50% to food energy intakes.

[†] The Dietary Reference Value for non-milk extrinsic sugars is that the population average intake should not exceed 11% of food energy intake.

[††] The Dietary Reference Value for total fat and saturated fatty acids is that the population average intake should not exceed 35% of food energy intake, and saturated fatty acids 11%.

18g/day than those aged 25 to 50 years, and women aged 19 to 24 years compared with those aged 35 to 50 years.

- The mean percentage of food energy derived from **total fat** was close to the DRV for each age and sex group (see Figure 3.2).
- The mean proportion of food energy derived from **saturated fatty acids** was above the DRV for each sex and age group (see Figure 3.3).

(Table 3.4; Figures 3.1 to 3.3)

3.2.3 Food sources of energy and macronutrients

Figures 3.4 to 3.7 show the percentage contribution of the major food types to mean daily intakes of total energy, total carbohydrate, non-milk extrinsic sugars, non-starch polysaccharides, total fat and saturated fatty acids.

Energy

Figure 3.4 shows that the main contributors to daily total energy intake were:

- cereals & cereal products, providing about one third of the average energy intake (31%);
- meat, meat dishes & meat products (15%);
- milk & milk products (10%); and
- drinks (10%).
- There were no significant sex or age differences in the contributions of the different food groups to total energy intake.

Figure 3.1

Mean daily intake of non-milk extrinsic sugars as percentage of food energy compared with Dietary Reference Value* by sex and age of respondent

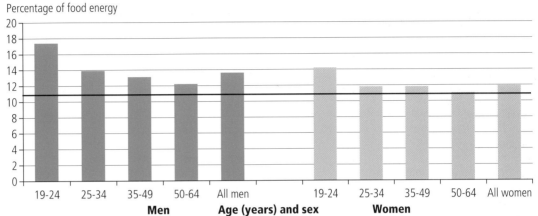

*   The current UK recommendation is that the population average intake of non-milk extrinsic sugars should not exceed 11% of food energy.

Figure 3.2

Mean daily intake of total fat as percentage of food energy compared with Dietary Reference Value* by sex and age of respondent

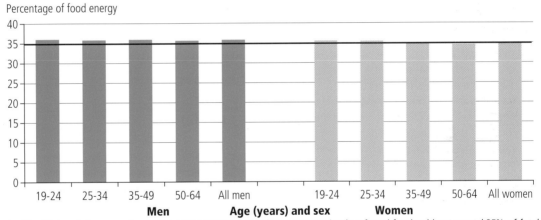

*   The Dietary Reference value for total fat is that the population average intake of total fat should not exceed 35% of food energy intake.

Figure 3.3

Mean daily intake of saturated fatty acids as percentage of food energy compared with Dietary Reference Value* by sex and age of respondent

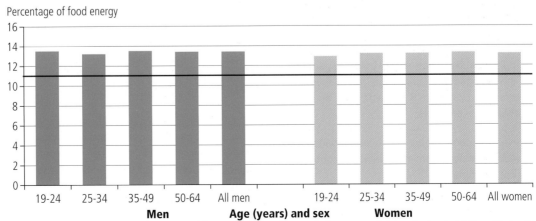

*   The Dietary Reference value for saturated fatty acids is that the population average intake of saturated fatty acids should not exceed 11% of food energy intake.

27

Total carbohydrate

Figure 3.4 also shows the main sources of total carbohydrate intake, these were:

- cereals & cereal products, contributing 45% to average total carbohydrate intake;
- potatoes (11%);
- drinks (10%); and
- sugar, preserves and confectionery (9%).
- There were no significant sex or age differences in the contributions of the different food groups to total carbohydrate intake.

Total fat and saturated fatty acids

Figure 3.5 shows that the main sources of total fat and saturated fatty acids in the diets of respondents were broadly similar. These were:

- meat, meat dishes & meat products, which contributed 23% to the intake of total fat and 22% to the intake of saturated fatty acids;
- cereals & cereal products, which accounted for almost a fifth, 19%, of the intake of total fat, and a similar proportion, 18%, of saturated fatty acids;
- milk & milk products, which provided 14% and 24% of total fat and saturated fatty acids intake respectively; and
- fat spreads, 12% and 11% respectively.
- Men obtained a higher proportion of their intake of saturated fatty acids from meat, meat dishes & meat products than women (data not shown, *see* Volume 3[5]).

Non-milk extrinsic sugars

As shown in Table 3.4, men and women in the youngest age group had higher mean intakes of non-milk extrinsic sugars than those in the oldest age group. Figures 3.6(a) and (b), therefore, show the main food types, and particular foods within these, that contributed most to total intakes of non-milk extrinsic sugars for all respondents aged 19 to 24 years compared with all respondents aged 50 to 64 years.

The main sources of non-milk extrinsic sugars for both the youngest and oldest age groups were: drinks; sugar, preserves & confectionery; and cereal & cereal products.

However, the contributions these foods made to non-milk extrinsic sugars intake differ according to age. For example:

- the main source of non-milk extrinsic sugars for the youngest group was drinks, which provided 57% of total intake (mainly from soft drinks, not low calorie) followed by sugar, preserves & confectionery (24%), whereas
- the main source of non-milk extrinsic sugars for the oldest group was sugar, preserves & confectionery (mainly table sugar), providing just over a third of total intake (34%) followed by drinks (27%).

Non-starch polysaccharides

Figure 3.7 shows the main food types, and particular foods within these, that contributed to total intake of non-starch polysaccharides. These were:

- cereals & cereal products, which accounted for 42% of total intake of non-starch polysaccharides. Within this group, breakfast cereals provided 13% of total intake and bread provided a further 20%;
- vegetables & vegetable dishes (excluding potatoes) which provided a fifth of total intake (20%);
- potatoes a further 13%; and
- fruit & nuts, 10%.

(Figures 3.4 to 3.7)

3.3 Alcohol

3.3.1 Introduction

For adults, sustained excessive consumption of alcohol has the effect of increasing the risk of high blood pressure and stroke. It is also a recognised risk factor for other conditions, for example cancers and cirrhosis of the liver[8].

Current recommendations, from the Department of Health[9], for alcohol consumption are:

- men should drink no more than three to four units of alcohol a day;
- women should drink no more than two to three units of alcohol a day.
- Heavy drinking is defined as consuming more than eight units a day for men and more than six a day for women.

A unit is defined as half a pint of beer, lager or cider, a 100ml glass of wine or one measure of spirits. Consistently drinking four or more units a day for men, or three or more units a day for women, is not advised as a sensible drinking level because of the progressive health risk it carries[9].

Figure 3.4

Percentage contribution of food types to average daily intake of total energy and carbohydrate: all respondents

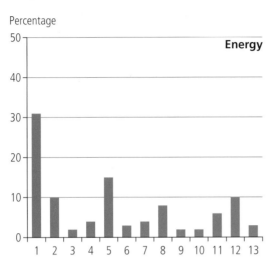

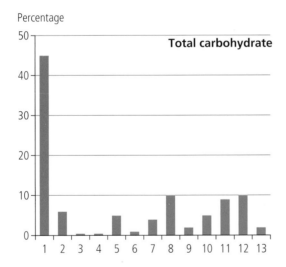

Figure 3.5

Percentage contribution of food types to average daily intake of total fat and saturated fatty acids: all respondents

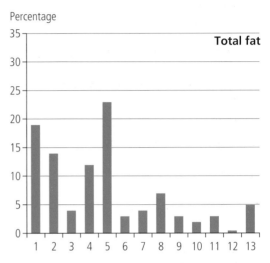

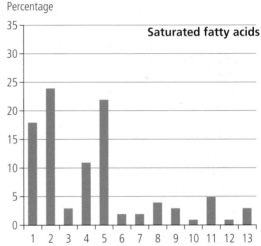

1	Cereals & cereal products
2	Milk & milk products
3	Eggs & egg dishes
4	Fat spreads
5	Meat, meat dishes & meat products
6	Fish & fish dishes
7	Vegetables & vegetable dishes (excluding potatoes)
8	Potatoes
9	Savoury snacks
10	Fruit & nuts
11	Sugar, preserves & confectionery
12	Drinks
13	Miscellaneous

1	Cereals & cereal products
2	Milk & milk products
3	Eggs & egg dishes
4	Fat spreads
5	Meat, meat dishes & meat products
6	Fish & fish dishes
7	Vegetables & vegetable dishes (excluding potatoes)
8	Potatoes
9	Savoury snacks
10	Fruit & nuts
11	Sugar, preserves & confectionery
12	Drinks
13	Miscellaneous

Figure 3.6(a)

Percentage contribution* of food types to average daily non-milk extrinsic sugars intake: all aged 19–24 years

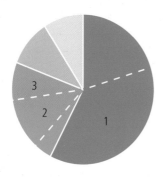

■ Drinks 57%
    Of which:
    ¹ Soft drinks, not low calorie (carbonated, concentrated, ready to drink) 37%

■ Sugar, preserves & confectionery 24%
    Of which:
    ² Table sugar 11%

    ³ Chocolate confectionery 8%

■ Cereals & cereal products 10%

■ Other** 9%

* All data are presented as a percentage of average daily total intake.
** Other includes: milk & milk products; eggs & egg dishes; fat spreads; meat, meat dishes & meat products; fish & fish dishes; vegetables & vegetable dishes (excluding potatoes); potatoes; savoury snacks; fruit & nuts; and miscellaneous.

Figure 3.6(b)

Percentage contribution* of food types to average daily non-milk extrinsic sugars intake: all aged 50–64 years

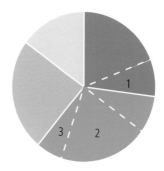

■ Drinks 27%
    Of which:
    ¹ Soft drinks, not low calorie (carbonated, concentrated, ready to drink) 8%

■ Sugar, preserves & confectionery 34%
    Of which:
    ² Table sugar 20%

    ³ Chocolate confectionery 6%

■ Cereals & cereal products 24%

■ Other** 15%

* All data are presented as a percentage of average daily total intake.
** Other includes: milk & milk products; eggs & egg dishes; fat spreads; meat, meat dishes & meat products; fish & fish dishes; vegetables & vegetable dishes (excluding potatoes); potatoes; savoury snacks; fruit & nuts; and miscellaneous.

Figure 3.7

Percentage contribution* of food types to average daily non-starch polysaccharides intake: all respondents

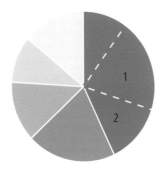

■ Cereals & cereal products 42%
   Of which:
   [1] Bread 20%

   [2] Breakfast cereals 13%

■ Vegetables & vegetable dishes (excluding potatoes) 20%

■ Potatoes 13%

■ Fruit & nuts 10%

□ Other** 14%

* All data are presented as a percentage of average daily total intake.

** Other includes: milk & milk products; eggs & egg dishes; fat spreads; meat, meat dishes & meat products; fish & fish dishes; savoury snacks; sugar, preserves & confectionery; drinks; and miscellaneous.

Information on alcohol consumption was collected as part of the dietary interview and also recorded in the seven-day dietary diary. Only information from the dietary diary is presented in this Volume. Data on alcohol consumption recorded as part of the dietary interview and analyses comparing the two sources are presented in Volume 2, Chapter 4[4,10]. Only alcohol from alcoholic drinks consumed was included in the comparison to daily benchmarks.

3.3.2 Alcohol consumption

Table 3.5 shows the mean number of units of alcohol consumed from alcoholic beverages during the seven-day dietary recording period, and the proportions consuming at or above the defined daily benchmarks, by sex and age. The latter was calculated for the day on which the respondent had consumed the most alcohol.

- Overall, and within each age group, men were more likely to consume alcohol than women, and consumed alcohol in greater quantities.
- 60% of men and 44% of women exceeded the recommendations for alcohol consumption on at least 1 day during the seven-day dietary recording period.
- Over a third of men, 39%, and over a fifth of women, 22%, drank heavily (that is, more than 8 units for men or 6 units for women) on their heaviest drinking day during the survey week.

By age:
- Men aged 35 to 49 years were more likely to exceed the recommendation for alcohol consumption compared with the oldest group of men.
- The youngest group of women were more likely to exceed the recommendation for alcohol consumption, and to drink heavily, than the oldest group of women.

(Table 3.5)

3.4 Vitamins and minerals

This section looks at mean daily intakes of vitamins and minerals from food sources, intakes compared with RNIs and LRNIs, and the percentage contribution of food types to intakes of these nutrients. The vitamins and minerals included are vitamin A, thiamin, riboflavin, niacin equivalents, vitamin B_6, vitamin B_{12}, folate, vitamin C, vitamin D, total iron, calcium, magnesium, potassium, zinc, iodine and copper[3]. More detailed information on these, and other vitamins and minerals not included in this Volume, can be found in Volume 3[5]. A brief explanation of the vitamins and minerals included in this section is given first.

3.4.1 Introduction

Vitamins

Vitamins are organic compounds, which are required in small amounts for growth, metabolism and health maintenance. They are essential substances which, with the exception of vitamin D, cannot be made within our bodies and therefore need to be obtained from our diet.

Vitamin A is essential for maintaining and repairing tissues needed for growth and normal development, and helps to maintain healthy skin and mucus linings such as in the nose. Vitamin A

Table 3.5

Maximum daily amount of alcohol consumed from alcoholic beverages (units) during seven-day dietary recording period by sex and age of respondent

Diary sample

Maximum daily amount*	Age of respondent (years):									All	
	19–24		25–34		35–49		50–64				
	%		%		%		%			%	
Men											
Drank nothing during last seven days	20		19		17		24			20	
Up to 4 units	14		19		18		24			20	
More than 4, up to 8 units	15	65	22	62	26	65	19	52		21	60
More than 8 units	50		40		40		33			39	
Mean number of units	9.4		8.3		8.2		6.3			7.8	
Base	*108*		*219*		*253*		*253*			*833*	
	%		%		%		%			%	
Women											
Drank nothing during last seven days	29		32		33		35			33	
Up to 3 units	14		21		23		29			23	
More than 3, up to 6 units	23	57	17	47**	23	44	22	36		21	44**
More than 6 units	34		29		21		14			22	
Mean number of units	5.3		4.0		3.6		2.7			3.6	
Base	*104*		*210*		*318*		*259*			*891*	

* Maximum daily amount is the number of units of alcohol consumed on the day on which the respondent had consumed most alcohol. Recommended daily benchmarks for men are no more than four units and for women no more than three units of alcohol. Heavy drinking is defined as more than eight units a day for men and six for women.

** In order to avoid rounding errors, the combined percentage has been calculated separately and may differ by one percentage point from the sum of the percentages in the individual categories.

also helps strengthen immunity from infections and is essential for vision in dim light. An early sign of vitamin A deficiency is night blindness.

B vitamins such as thiamin (vitamin B_1), riboflavin (vitamin B_2), niacin (or nicotinic acid), vitamin B_6 and vitamin B_{12}, have several features in common, although the chemical structure of each of these B-vitamins is quite different. They act as 'co-factors' in different enzyme systems in the body. Between them, these vitamins are necessary for the metabolism of protein and fat, the release and utilisation of energy from food, the formation of new cells including healthy red blood cells, and to ensure a healthy nervous system.

Folate (or folic acid) is needed by the body to make DNA, for the formation of new cells and the production of healthy red blood cells. An optimal intake of folate both prior to conception and during pregnancy is particularly important. Research has shown that women who increase their folate intake before pregnancy and during its early stages can help to reduce their risk of having a child with a neural tube defect (NTD) such as spina bifida. This is where the brain or spinal cord or their protective coverings fail to develop properly. It is therefore recommended that, to reduce the risk of NTDs in the unborn child, all women who could become pregnant take a 400 microgram folic acid supplement daily prior to conception until the 12th week of pregnancy[11].

Vitamin C is needed for the maintenance of healthy connective tissue in the body, acts as an antioxidant protecting cells from the damage caused by free radicals, and helps in the absorption of iron. Deficiency soon results in bleeding, especially from small blood vessels under the skin and from the gums, and prolonged healing times for wounds.

Vitamin D is essential for healthy bones and teeth and helps to maintain bone mineralisation primarily by enhancing the absorption of dietary calcium. It is also important for a healthy nervous system and muscle function. Vitamin D is obtained both from the action of sunlight on the skin and from the diet. For most people, sunlight is the most important source and little or no extra will be needed from food. Adequate summer exposure to sunlight provides sufficient vitamin D stores throughout winter. Food sources are therefore particularly important for those who do not receive adequate sunlight, and also for children and pregnant and lactating women. Vitamin D is found naturally in some animal products, including oily fish. Some foods, such as margarine and fat spreads, and some breakfast cereals, are fortified with vitamin D.

Minerals

Minerals are inorganic elements. Some minerals are required for the body's normal function and these essential minerals are obtained from the diet and include iron, calcium, potassium, magnesium, sodium and chloride. Trace elements are required in minute amounts, and include zinc, copper and iodine.

Iron is an integral part of haemoglobin, found in red blood cells. It plays a major role in the body's use of oxygen, transporting oxygen from the lungs to the cells of the body. Other iron-containing molecules utilise oxygen within the cells.

Calcium is the most abundant mineral in the body and is vital for healthy bones and teeth. It is also essential for muscle contraction (including heart muscle), nerve function, the activity of several enzymes and for normal blood clotting. Vitamin D is extremely important for the absorption of calcium in the body.

Potassium is necessary for maintaining fluid and electrolyte balance in the body cells and has a complementary action with sodium in the functioning of cells. The potassium inside the cells balances the sodium outside the cells to maintain pressure and water balance in the body.

Most of the *magnesium* in the body is present in bones and it is thought to have a function in bone health. It is also an essential constituent of all cells and is involved in a large number of metabolic processes, including the functioning of some of the enzymes which are involved in energy utilisation.

Trace elements include *zinc*, *iodine* and *copper*. *Zinc* is a component of a wide variety of enzymes and is involved with a number of metabolic processes. It is required to release energy from food, for a normal sense of taste and smell, and for the normal growth and regeneration of new cells and wound healing. Zinc is also essential for immune defence systems within the body. *Iodine* is an essential constituent of hormones produced by the thyroid gland which control metabolism and are essential for normal growth and development. *Copper* is associated with a number of enzymes within the body, and has an important role in many chemical reactions to ensure good health. Research suggests that adequate status is needed to maintain antioxidant defences.

3.4.2 Intakes of vitamins and minerals

Table 3.6 shows mean (average) daily intakes of the above vitamins and minerals from food sources, that is, excluding intakes from dietary supplements, by sex and age. These intakes are also compared with the RNI for each nutrient (no RNIs have been set for vitamin D for adults aged 19 to 64 years)[12]. The proportion of adults with intakes below the LRNI is shown in Table 3.7. To

ensure that the risk of deficiency within a group is very small, the average group intake of a nutrient should be at or above the RNI, which is the amount that is sufficient, or more than sufficient, for about 97% of the people in a group. The LRNI for a vitamin or mineral is the amount of that nutrient which is enough for only a few people in a group with low needs[6].

- Both men and women in the youngest age group had lower mean intakes of many of these vitamins and minerals compared with those in the oldest age group.

Comparing mean daily intakes of these vitamins and minerals to the appropriate RNI, Table 3.6 shows that:

- Mean (average) intakes of all vitamins presented were close to the RNI for all sex/age groups except for vitamin A in the youngest groups of men and women.
- Mean intakes of all minerals presented were below the RNI for a number of sex/age groups. For example:
  - For men, mean intakes of potassium and magnesium were well below the RNI for the youngest group.
  - For women, mean intakes of magnesium, potassium and copper were below the RNI for all age groups and intakes of iron were well below the RNI in all but the oldest group.

Table 3.7 shows the proportion of men and women, by age, with low intakes of vitamins and minerals from food sources, that is, intakes below the LRNI. In general, a higher proportion of the youngest group of women and, to a lesser extent the youngest group of men, had low intakes of vitamins and minerals compared with the oldest group.

- There was evidence of low intakes of vitamin A, riboflavin, magnesium and potassium, for men and women, particularly in the youngest age groups, and of iodine in the youngest group of women.
- There was evidence of low intakes of iron in women. Over 40% of the two youngest age groups had low intakes.

The proportion of respondents with intakes of iron below the LRNI is also shown in Figure 3.8. Iron requirements are set higher for women than men, and higher for women aged 19 to 50 years than for those aged over 50 years, to take account of menstrual losses. No more than 3% of men in any age group had a mean daily intake of total iron, from food sources, below the LRNI. However, a

Table 3.6

Average daily intake of vitamins and minerals (from food sources, that is excluding dietary supplements) and average daily intakes as a percentage of the Reference Nutrient Intake (RNI) by sex and age of respondent

Vitamins and minerals	Men aged (years):				All men	Women aged (years):				All women
	19–24	25–34	35–49	50–64		19–24	25–34	35–49	50–64	
Vitamins										
Vitamin A (retinol equivalents) (µg)										
Mean (average value)	560	724	989	1145	911	467	587	675	816	671
% of RNI*	80%	103%	141%	164%	130%	78%	98%	112%	136%	112%
Thiamin (mg)										
Mean (average value)	1.60	2.08	2.04	2.07	2.00	1.45	1.55	1.52	1.60	1.54
% of RNI*	160%	232%	204%	230%	214%	181%	194%	190%	200%	193%
Riboflavin (mg)										
Mean (average value)	1.68	2.12	2.19	2.20	2.11	1.39	1.44	1.66	1.75	1.60
% of RNI*	129%	163%	168%	169%	162%	126%	131%	151%	159%	146%
Niacin equivalents (mg)										
Mean (average value)	39.4	46.2	45.9	44.6	44.7	29.5	28.8	31.5	32.3	30.9
% of RNI*	232%	272%	270%	279%	268%	246%	240%	263%	270%	257%
Vitamin B_6 (mg)										
Mean (average value)	2.6	3.0	2.9	2.8	2.9	2.0	1.9	2.0	2.1	2.0
% of RNI*	189%	211%	206%	201%	204%	165%	158%	170%	177%	169%
Vitamin B_{12} (µg)										
Mean (average value)	4.4	5.9	7.0	7.3	6.5	4.0	4.0	4.9	5.7	4.8
% of RNI*	296%	395%	465%	485%	431%	266%	264%	325%	378%	319%
Folate (µg)										
Mean (average value)	301	346	343	361	344	229	234	255	268	251
% of RNI*	151%	173%	171%	181%	172%	114%	117%	128%	134%	125%
Vitamin C (mg)										
Mean (average value)	64.9	74.1	88.4	94.5	83.4	67.9	72.3	80.0	94.5	81.0
% of RNI*	162%	185%	221%	236%	209%	170%	181%	200%	236%	202%
Vitamin D (µg)**										
Mean (average value)	2.9	3.5	3.7	4.2	3.7	2.3	2.4	2.8	3.5	2.8
Base	*108*	*219*	*253*	*253*	*833*	*104*	*210*	*318*	*259*	*891*
Minerals										
Total iron (mg)										
Mean (average value)	11.4	13.0	13.7	13.6	13.2	8.8	9.2	10.2	10.9	10.0
% of RNI*	131%	150%	157%	156%	151%	60%	62%	69%	122%	82%
Calcium (mg)										
Mean (average value)	860	1017	1040	1027	1007	694	731	796	823	777
% of RNI*	123%	145%	149%	147%	144%	99%	104%	114%	118%	111%
Magnesium (mg)										
Mean (average value)	258	308	318	318	308	205	209	235	246	229
% of RNI*	86%	103%	106%	106%	103%	76%	77%	87%	91%	85%
Potassium (mg)										
Mean (average value)	2841	3284	3481	3552	3367	2362	2397	2731	2884	2653
% of RNI*	81%	94%	99%	101%	96%	67%	68%	78%	82%	76%
Zinc (mg)										
Mean (average value)	9.0	10.2	10.6	10.3	10.2	6.8	6.7	7.6	7.8	7.4
% of RNI*	95%	108%	111%	109%	107%	98%	96%	108%	112%	105%
Iodine (µg)										
Mean (average value)	166	216	221	230	215	130	145	162	178	159
% of RNI*	119%	154%	158%	164%	154%	93%	103%	116%	127%	114%
Copper (mg)										
Mean (average value)	1.14	1.37	1.53	1.51	1.43	0.91	1.00	1.05	1.07	1.03
% of RNI*	95%	114%	128%	126%	119%	76%	83%	88%	89%	86%
Base	*108*	*219*	*253*	*253*	*833*	*104*	*210*	*318*	*259*	*891*

*   Intake as a percentage of RNI was calculated for each respondent. The values for all respondents in each age group were then pooled to give a mean value.

**   No RNIs have been set for vitamin D for adults. Vitamin D is obtained both from the action of sunlight on the skin, and from the diet.

Table 3.7

Proportion of respondents with average daily intakes (from food sources, that is excluding dietary supplements) of vitamins and minerals below the Lower Reference Nutrient Intake (LRNI) by sex and age of respondent

Vitamins and minerals	% with average daily intake below the LRNI									
	Men aged (years):				All men	Women aged (years):				All women
	19–24	25–34	35–49	50–64		19–24	25–34	35–49	50–64	
Vitamins*										
Vitamin A	16	7	5	4	7	19	11	8	5	9
Thiamin	2	0	0	1	1	-	2	1	1	1
Riboflavin	8	1	2	3	3	15	10	5	6	8
Niacin equivalents	-	-	0	0	0	2	-	1	0	1
Vitamin B_6	-	0	2	1	1	5	1	2	2	2
Vitamin B_{12}	1	-	0	0	0	1	1	1	0	1
Folate	2	-	0	-	0	3	2	2	2	2
Vitamin C	-	0	-	-	0	1	-	0	0	0
Base	*108*	*219*	*253*	*253*	*833*	*104*	*210*	*318*	*259*	*891*
Minerals*										
Total iron	3	0	1	1	1	42	41	27	4	25
Calcium	5	2	2	2	2	8	6	6	3	5
Magnesium	17	9	7	9	9	22	20	10	7	13
Potassium	18	3	5	5	6	30	30	16	10	19
Zinc	7	2	4	3	4	5	5	4	3	4
Iodine	2	1	2	1	2	12	5	4	1	4
Base	*108*	*219*	*253*	*253*	*833*	*104*	*210*	*318*	*259*	*891*

* There are no LRNIs for vitamin D and copper, and these nutrients do not appear in this table.

Figure 3.8

Proportion of respondents with average daily intakes of iron (from food sources, that is excluding dietary supplements) below the Lower Reference Nutrient Intake (LRNI)* by sex and age of respondent

Percentage below LRNI

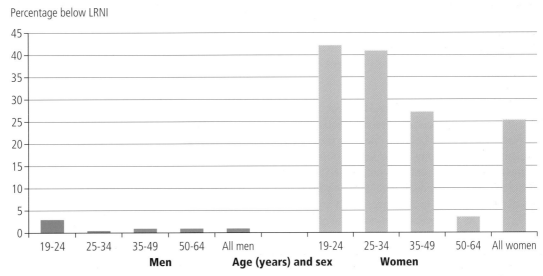

* LRNIs for iron are set at 4.7mg/d for men, 8.0mg/d for women aged 19 to 50 years and 4.7mg/d for women over the age of 50.

quarter of women overall, 25%, over 40% of those aged 19 to 34 years and over a quarter, 27%, of those aged 35 to 49 years had low iron intakes.

(Tables 3.6 and 3.7, Figure 3.8)

3.4.3 Dietary supplements

In Chapter 2 it was shown that 35% of respondents reported taking dietary supplements. The effect of dietary supplements on intakes of vitamins and minerals is considered in the following section (data taken from Volume 3[5]).

Dietary supplements increased mean intakes of vitamin A, thiamin, riboflavin, vitamin B_6, vitamin B_{12}, folate, vitamin C, vitamin D, iron, and zinc for men and women overall by between 4% and 45%. For these nutrients, dietary supplements made a greater contribution to mean intakes for women than for men, and there were also differences by age in the contribution of supplements to mean intakes. For example, mean daily intake of vitamin D for women aged 50 to 64 years increased by 46% when dietary supplements were included. However, for all these nutrients except vitamin A and iron, mean intakes *from food sources only*, for all sex and age groups were already close to, or above, the RNI.

Dietary supplements increased mean daily intakes of:

- vitamin A to close to the RNI for women aged 19 to 24 years. However, vitamin A intakes remained well below the RNI for men aged 19 to 24 years even when dietary supplements were included; and
- total iron as a percentage of the RNI for all sex/age groups, but mean intakes including supplements for women aged 19 to 49 years were still well below the RNI.

Dietary supplements had little effect on the number of people with low intakes of these vitamins and minerals.

The LRNI for folate is 100µg/day. However, the Department of Health currently recommends that women who could become pregnant take a supplement of 400µg/day of folic acid in order to minimise the risk of neural tube defects (NTD)[11]. In this survey, 86% of women aged 19 to 24 years, 92% of those aged 25 to 34 years and 84% of women aged 35 to 49 years had an intake of folate from all sources, including supplements containing folic acid, of less than 400µg/day.

3.4.4 Food sources of vitamins and minerals

Figures 3.9 to 3.14 show the percentage contribution of major food types, and particular foods within these, to mean daily intakes of selected vitamins and minerals. More detailed information on the food sources of these vitamins and minerals can be found in Volume 3[5].

Food sources of vitamin A

Tables 3.6 and 3.7 showed that mean intakes of vitamin A were below the RNI for the youngest group of men and for women aged 19 to 34 years, and that the proportion with low intakes was higher in the youngest age groups. The contribution of foods to intakes of vitamin A are, therefore, shown for men and women aged 19 to 24 years and men and women aged 50 to 64 years (Figures 3.9(a) to (d)).

Overall, the main food sources of vitamin A were: meat, meat dishes & meat products (in particular liver, liver products & dishes); vegetables & vegetable dishes (excluding potatoes) (in particular carrots); milk & milk products; and fat spreads. Liver and carrots are rich sources of vitamin A.

The contribution made by these groups differed by sex and age, such that:

- meat, meat dishes & meat products, particularly liver, liver products & dishes, were the main source of vitamin A for men overall, whereas for women overall, the main source was vegetables & vegetable dishes (excluding potatoes) (data not shown, *see* Volume 3[5]);
- meat, meat dishes & meat products made a lower contribution to total vitamin A intake for the youngest group of men compared with those in the oldest group, whereas contributions from vegetables & vegetable dishes (excluding potatoes), milk & milk products and fat spreads were similar; and
- within the meat, meat dishes & meat products group, the contribution made by liver, liver products & dishes increased significantly with age for both sexes.

Food sources of vitamin C

Figures 3.10(a) and (b) show the differences in the contributions made by the main food sources of vitamin C for all respondents aged 19 to 24 years and all respondents aged 50 to 64 years.

The main sources of vitamin C intake were: drinks, in particular fruit juice and certain soft drinks; vegetables & vegetable dishes (excluding potatoes); potatoes; and fruit (excluding fruit juice).

However:

- The youngest group obtained a higher proportion of their total vitamin C intake from drinks, 40%, than the oldest group, 22%, and a lower proportion from vegetables & vegetable dishes (excluding potatoes), 13% compared with 25%, and fruit (excluding fruit juice), 9% compared with 24%.
- Men derived a significantly lower proportion of their vitamin C intake from fruit (excluding fruit juice) than women, 16% compared with 22% (data not shown, *see* Volume 3[5]).

Food sources of vitamin D

As shown in Chapter 4, men in the youngest age group had lower concentrations of vitamin D in the blood than the oldest group of men. Therefore, Figures 3.11(a) to (d) show the main food sources of vitamin D for the youngest and oldest group of men and women. It should be noted that diet is not the only source of vitamin D, as it is also obtained through the action of sunlight on the skin.

The main sources of vitamin D in the diets of respondents in this survey were: cereals & cereal products (in particular fortified breakfast cereals); fat spreads; meat, meat dishes & meat products; and fish & fish dishes.

Nearly all the contribution from fish & fish dishes came from oily fish, which is a rich source of vitamin D. Some breakfast cereals are fortified with vitamin D, and vitamin D is required by law to be added to margarine, and is also added to most reduced and low fat spreads.

- The youngest men and women obtained a lower proportion of their total vitamin D intake from fish & fish dishes (that is, oily fish) compared with the oldest group (3% and 21% compared with 28% and 37% respectively).
- Overall, men obtained more of their vitamin D intake from meat, meat dishes & meat products than women, whereas women obtained more of their vitamin D intake from oily fish (data not shown, *see* Volume 3[5]).

Food sources of folate

Figure 3.12 shows that the main source of folate in the diets of respondents were:

- cereals & cereal products, providing a third, 33%, of mean daily intake overall, of which just under half, 15%, came from breakfast cereals, many of which are fortified with folate;
- vegetables & vegetable dishes (excluding potatoes) (15%);
- drinks (14%); and
- potatoes (11%).
- There were no significant age differences for men or women in the contribution of food groups to average daily intake of folate.

Food sources of total iron

Some foods are fortified with iron, for example flour and many breakfast cereals. All wheat flour, other than wholemeal flour, is fortified with iron by law; other foods are not subject to compulsory fortification but are fortified voluntarily by manufacturers. Thus, cereals & cereal products were found to be the major source of iron for respondents in this survey (Figure 3.12).

- Overall, respondents obtained over two-fifths, 44%, of mean daily intake of total iron from cereals & cereal products. Within this group the major sources were breakfast cereals, providing 20% of mean total iron intake overall, and white bread, contributing 9% overall;
- meat, meat dishes & meat products (17%); and
- vegetables & vegetable dishes (excluding potatoes) (10%).
- There were no significant sex or age differences in the contributions of the different food groups to iron intake.

Food sources of magnesium

Figure 3.12 shows the main food sources of magnesium for all respondents were:

- cereals & cereal products, providing just over one quarter, 27%, of mean intake overall, about half of which, 13%, came from bread;
- drinks (17%);
- meat, meat dishes & meat products (12%); and
- milk & milk products (11%).
- There were no significant differences by age in the contribution of food groups to mean daily intake of magnesium.

Food sources of calcium[13]

Figure 3.13 shows the main food sources of calcium for all respondents. These were:

- milk & milk products, contributing 43% to mean intake overall. Within this group, milk (whole, semi-skimmed, skimmed) and cheese were the main contributors, providing 27% and 11% respectively; and
- cereals & cereal products (30%). White flour is fortified with calcium. Over a third of the contribution from cereals & cereal products came from white bread, 13%.
- There were no significant differences by sex or age in the proportion of mean daily calcium intake accounted for by the different food groups.

Food sources of potassium

Figure 3.14 shows the main food sources of potassium for all respondents. These were:

- potatoes, with respondents, overall, obtaining 16% of their mean intake of potassium from this source;
- drinks (15%), including 5% for men and, significantly lower, 1% for women from beer & lager;
- meat, meat dishes & meat products (15%) ;
- milk & milk products (13%);
- cereals & cereal products (13%); and
- vegetables & vegetable dishes (excluding potatoes) (10%).
- There were no significant differences by age in the contributions of the different food groups to potassium intake.

Food sources of zinc

Figure 3.14 also shows the main food sources of zinc for all respondents. These were:

- meat, meat dishes & meat products, which provided about a third, 34%, of the mean daily intake of zinc;
- cereals & cereal products, 25%; and
- milk & milk products (17%).
- There were no significant sex or age differences in the contribution of food groups to mean daily intake of zinc.

Food sources of copper

Figure 3.14 also shows the main food sources of copper for all respondents were:

- cereals & cereal products, accounting for about a third, 31% of intake;
- meat, meat dishes & meat products (15%);
- fruit & nuts (10%);
- potatoes (9%); and
- drinks (9%).

- Meat, meat dishes & meat products accounted for a higher proportion of copper intake for men than for women (data not shown).
- There were no significant differences by age in the contribution of food groups to mean daily copper intake.

(Figures 3.9 to 3.14)

3.4.5 Salt

Salt is made up of two elements, sodium and chloride. Sodium is a vital component of the body and thus is an essential nutrient. It is involved in maintaining the water balance of the body and is essential for muscle and nerve activity. All fluids within the body contain salt (that is, sodium chloride), especially those fluids outside the cells such as blood.

A habitually higher intake of salt has been linked to a higher than average blood pressure, which may lead to an increased risk of heart disease or a stroke. A diet lower in salt would be expected to result in lower average blood pressure and a smaller rise in blood pressure with age. Other lifestyle factors that also affect blood pressure include body weight, alcohol consumption and physical activity.

In the Report on Nutritional Aspects of Cardiovascular Disease, the Committee on Medical Aspects of Food Policy (COMA) recommended:

- an intake of salt of 6g/day or less[14].

This recommendation was endorsed by the Scientific Advisory Committee on Nutrition in its recent report 'Salt and Health'[15].

This section looks at self-reported use of salt as reported in the dietary interview, average salt intakes[16] and the main food sources of sodium in the diets of respondents to this survey. Data from the current survey are also compared to data from the 1986/87 Adults Survey[2].

Use of Salt

Respondents were asked, during the dietary interview, whether salt is used in cooking their food and whether they add salt to their food at the table. These questions asked about frequency of use, rather than how much salt was used.

- Almost three quarters of all respondents, 73%, reported that salt was usually added to their food during cooking[17].

NDNS adults aged 19 to 64, Volume 5 2004

Figure 3.9(a)

Percentage contribution* of food types to average daily intake of vitamin A (retinol equivalents): men aged 19–24 years

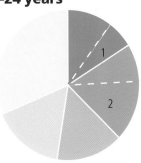

- Meat, meat dishes & meat products 16%
  Of which:
  [1] Liver, liver products & dishes 6%

- Vegetables & vegetable dishes (excluding potatoes) 21%
  Of which:
  [2] Carrots (raw, not raw) 13%

- Milk & milk products 15%

- Fat spreads 16%

- Other** 31%

Figure 3.9(b)

Percentage contribution* of food types to average daily intake of vitamin A (retinol equivalents): men aged 50–64 years

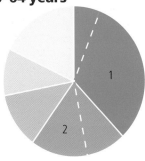

- Meat, meat dishes & meat products 38%
  Of which:
  [1] Liver, liver products & dishes 32%

- Vegetables & vegetable dishes (excluding potatoes) 23%
  Of which:
  [2] Carrots (raw, not raw) 13%

- Milk & milk products 12%

- Fat spreads 10%

- Other** 18%

Figure 3.9(c)

Percentage contribution* of food types to average daily intake of vitamin A (retinol equivalents): women aged 19–24 years

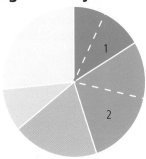

- Meat, meat dishes & meat products 16%
  Of which:
  [1] Liver, liver products & dishes 9%

- Vegetables & vegetable dishes (excluding potatoes) 28%
  Of which:
  [2] Carrots (raw, not raw) 16%

- Milk & milk products 19%

- Fat spreads 9%

- Other** 26%

Figure 3.9(d)

Percentage contribution* of food types to average daily intake of vitamin A (retinol equivalents): women aged 50–64 years

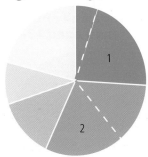

- Meat, meat dishes & meat products 26%
  Of which:
  [1] Liver, liver products & dishes 21%

- Vegetables & vegetable dishes (excluding potatoes) 31%
  Of which:
  [2] Carrots (raw, not raw) 18%

- Milk & milk products 13%

- Fat spreads 9%

- Other** 21%

* All data are presented as a percentage of average daily total intake.

** Other includes: cereals & cereal products; eggs & egg dishes; fish & fish dishes; potatoes; savoury snacks; fruit & nuts; sugar, preserves & confectionery; drinks; and miscellaneous.

Figure 3.10(a)

Percentage contribution* of food types to average daily vitamin C intake: all aged 19–24 years

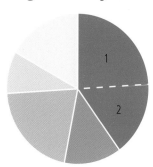

- Drinks 40%
  Of which:
  [1] Fruit juice 24%

  [2] Soft drinks 16%

- Vegetables & vegetable dishes (excluding potatoes) 13%

- Potatoes 21%

- Fruit (excluding fruit juice) 9%

- Other** 17%

Figure 3.10(b)

Percentage contribution* of food types to average daily vitamin C intake: all aged 50–64 years

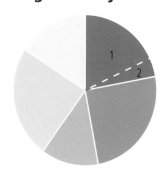

- Drinks 22%
  Of which:
  [1] Fruit juice 18%

  [2] Soft drinks 4%

- Vegetables & vegetable dishes (excluding potatoes) 25%

- Potatoes 13%

- Fruit (excluding fruit juice) 24%

- Other** 16%

*   All data are presented as a percentage of average daily total intake.
** Other includes: cereals & cereal products; milk & milk products; eggs & egg dishes; fat spreads; meat, meat dishes & meat products fish & fish dishes; savoury snacks; nuts; sugar, preserves & confectionery; drinks; and miscellaneous.

Figure 3.11(a)

Percentage contribution* of food types to average daily intake of vitamin D**: men aged 19–24 years

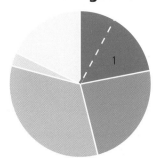

- Cereals & cereal products 22%
  Of which:
  [1] Breakfast cereals 14%

- Fat spreads 24%

- Meat, meat dishes & meat products 33%

- Fish & fish dishes*** 3%

- Other**** 18%

Figure 3.11(b)

Percentage contribution* of food types to average daily intake of vitamin D**: men aged 50–64 years

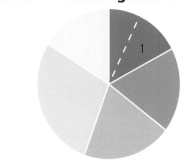

- Cereals & cereal products 17%
  Of which:
  [1] Breakfast cereals 10%

- Fat spreads 18%

- Meat, meat dishes & meat products 20%

- Fish & fish dishes*** 28%

- Other**** 16%

Figure 3.11(c)

Percentage contribution of food types to average daily intake of vitamin D****: women aged 19–24 years**

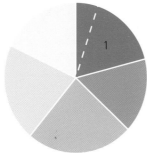

■ Cereals & cereal products 21%
    Of which:
    ¹ Breakfast cereals 16%

■ Fat spreads 16%

■ Meat, meat dishes & meat products 24%

■ Fish & fish dishes*** 21%

  Other**** 18%

Figure 3.11(d)

Percentage contribution of food types to average daily intake of vitamin D****: women aged 50–64 years**

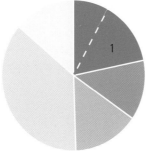

■ Cereals & cereal products 22%
    Of which:
    ¹ Breakfast cereals 14%

■ Fat spreads 13%

■ Meat, meat dishes & meat products 15%

■ Fish & fish dishes*** 37%

  Other**** 14%

*   *All data are presented as a percentage of average daily total intake.*

**   *Diet is not the only source of vitamin D, vitamin D is also obtained from the action of sunlight on the skin.*

*** *Nearly all the contribution from 'fish & fish dishes' came from oily fish, which is a rich source of vitamin D.*

**** *Other includes: milk & milk products; eggs & egg dishes; vegetables & vegetable dishes (excluding potatoes); potatoes; savoury snacks; fruit & nuts; sugar, preserves & confectionery; drinks; and miscellaneous.*

Figure 3.12

Percentage contribution of food types to average daily intake of folate, iron and magnesium: all respondents

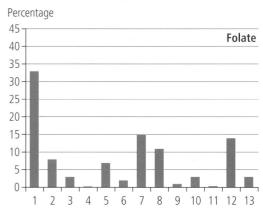

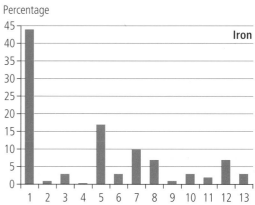

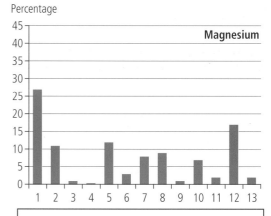

1	Cereals & cereal products
2	Milk & milk products
3	Eggs & egg dishes
4	Fat spreads
5	Meat, meat dishes & meat products
6	Fish & fish dishes
7	Vegetables & vegetable dishes (excluding potatoes)
8	Potatoes
9	Savoury snacks
10	Fruit & nuts
11	Sugar, preserves & confectionery
12	Drinks
13	Miscellaneous

Figure 3.13

Percentage contribution* of food types to average daily intake of calcium: all respondents

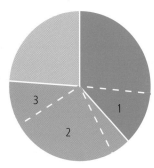

■ Cereals & cereal products 30%
  Of which:
    ¹ White bread 13%

■ Milk & milk products 43%
  Of which:
    ² Milk (whole, semi-skimmed, skimmed) 27%

    ³ Cheese 11%

■ Other** 27%

* All data are presented as a percentage of average daily total intake.
** Other includes: eggs & egg dishes; fat spreads; meat, meat dishes & meat products; fish & fish dishes; vegetables & vegetable dishes (excluding potatoes); potatoes; savoury snacks; fruit & nuts; sugar, preserves & confectionery; drinks; and miscellaneous.

Figure 3.14

Percentage contribution of food types to average daily intake of potassium, zinc and copper: all respondents

Percentage

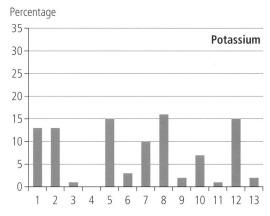

Percentage

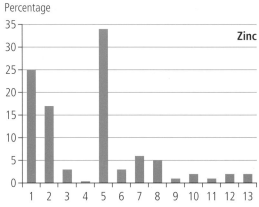

Percentage

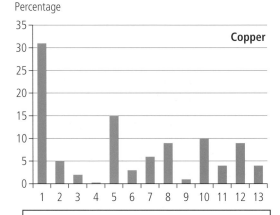

1	Cereals & cereal products
2	Milk & milk products
3	Eggs & egg dishes
4	Fat spreads
5	Meat, meat dishes & meat products
6	Fish & fish dishes
7	Vegetables & vegetable dishes (excluding potatoes)
8	Potatoes
9	Savoury snacks
10	Fruit & nuts
11	Sugar, preserves & confectionery
12	Drinks
13	Miscellaneous

- Men were more likely than women to report adding salt to their food at the table, either 'usually' or 'occasionally', 61% compared with 51%. Women were more likely than men to say that they never added salt at the table, 30% compared with 24%.

There were no clear age patterns in the use of salt in cooking or at the table.

Table 3.8 shows mean salt intakes calculated from analysis of respondents' urine samples, collected over a 24-hour period[16]. This analysis is important as dietary estimates exclude salt added at the table and in cooking, and so underestimate total intake. Figure 3.15 shows mean daily intakes of salt compared with the daily recommended value of 6g.

- Mean intakes exceeded the 6g per day recommendation in all sex/age groups, and were higher for men (11.0g/day) compared with women (8.1g/day).
- 15% of men and 31% of women had salt intakes of 6g per day or less, on average, over the survey week.
- There were no significant differences in mean salt intakes by age for men or women.
- Mean salt intake for men and women is slightly higher in the current survey, 9.5g/day, compared with 9g/day in the 1986/87 Adults Survey[2].

(Table 3.8, Figure 3.15)

Food sources of sodium[18]

Figure 3.16 shows the main food sources of sodium for all respondents were:

- cereals & cereal products, providing over one third, 35%, of mean intake overall, with white bread alone providing 14% of mean daily intake, breakfast cereals 5%, and biscuits, buns, cakes & pastries 4%;
- meat, meat dishes & meat products provided a further 26% overall, with bacon & ham, contributing 8%, and chicken, turkey & dishes, including coated chicken, providing 5%;
- milk & milk products (8%); and
- vegetables & vegetable dishes (excluding potatoes) (7%).
- There were no significant sex or age differences in the contribution of food groups to mean daily intake of sodium.

(Figure 3.16)

3.5 Variation in nutrient intake by region and household receipt of benefits

This section looks at differences in mean daily intakes of energy, total carbohydrate, non-milk extrinsic sugars, non-starch polysaccharides, total fat, saturated fatty acids, and selected vitamins and minerals from food sources (that is, excluding dietary supplements) by region and household receipt of benefits. For more detailed information on differences by these variables, *see* Volumes 2 and 3[4,5].

3.5.1 Region[19]

Overall, there were few clear differences in intakes of energy, macronutrients, vitamins and minerals between the four different regions. This is in line with the finding that there were no consistent differences between the regions in patterns of food consumption (*see* Chapter 2).

However, women in London and the South East met the recommendation of 11% of food energy derived from non-milk extrinsic sugars, and men in all regions and women in all other regions exceeded the recommendation.

- For all vitamins, mean daily intake from food sources was above the RNI for men and women in each of the four regions. For those minerals where mean daily intakes were below the RNI for the group as a whole, the same was true for all regions.
- There were no significant regional differences in the proportion of men or women with intakes from food sources below the LRNI for any of the vitamins.
- Women in Scotland were less likely to have an intake of iodine below the LRNI than women in any other region.

3.5.2 Household receipt of benefits[20]

Adults living in households in receipt of benefits had lower average intake of energy and some nutrients, particularly vitamins and minerals, compared with adults in non-benefit households. Both men and women living in households in receipt of benefits had lower mean daily total energy intake than those in non-benefit households, which resulted in lower absolute intakes of some macronutrients.

However, when intakes are expressed as a percentage of energy intake, to account for differences in energy intakes, the results show that women in benefit households obtained a

Table 3.8

Percentage distribution of salt intake (g/day) estimated from total urinary sodium by sex and age of respondent

*Respondents who reported making a full 24-hour urine collection**

Salt intake (g/day)	Men aged (years):				All men	Women aged (years):				All women
	19–24	25–34	35–49	50–64		19–24	25–34	35–49	50–64	
	cum %	cum %	cum %	cum %	cum %	cum %	cum %	cum %	cum %	cum %
3 or less	-	5	2	5	4	4	6	5	7	6
6 or less	2	20	13	18	15	17	29	31	38	31
9 or less	37	34	39	42	39	66	59	68	69	66
12 or less	60	57	58	65	60	84	81	85	91	86
15 or less	81	73	80	83	79	90	92	96	96	95
18 or less	100	89	91	91	91	92	97	100	99	98
All		100	100	100	100	100	100		100	100
Base	62	152	170	183	567	60	129	203	187	580
Mean	11.0	11.4	11.1	10.5	11.0	9.1	8.7	8.0	7.5	8.1
Median	10.6	10.9	10.2	10.1	10.4	7.6	8.0	7.5	7.0	7.6
Lower 2.5 percentile	6.0	2.2	2.4	2.1	2.4	1.7	1.9	2.6	2.3	2.3
Upper 2.5 percentile	16.6	22.3	22.1	21.2	21.6	23.2	22.2	16.2	15.7	16.5
Standard deviation	3.41	5.79	4.83	4.95	5.02	4.62	4.61	3.42	3.45	3.88

* This excludes 298 cases where the respondent reported missing at least one collection.

Figure 3.15

Mean daily intake of salt (g/day) compared with COMA recommendation* by sex and age of respondent

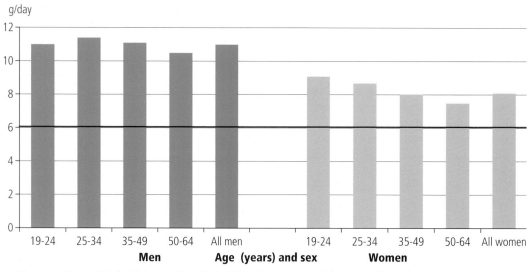

* The Committee on Medical Aspects of Food Policy (COMA) recommended an intake of salt of 6g/day or less.

Figure 3.16

Percentage contribution of food types to average daily intake of sodium: all respondents*

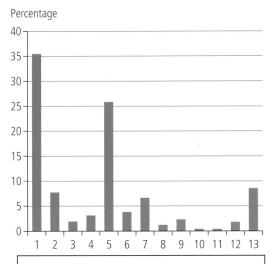

Percentage

1	Cereals & cereal products
2	Milk & milk products
3	Eggs & egg dishes
4	Fat spreads
5	Meat, meat dishes & meat products
6	Fish & fish dishes
7	Vegetables & vegetable dishes (excluding potatoes)
8	Potatoes
9	Savoury snacks
10	Fruit & nuts
11	Sugar, preserves & confectionery
12	Drinks
13	Miscellaneous

* Data in this table are for intakes from food only and do not include further additions of salt in cooking or at the table.

higher proportion of their energy intake from non-milk extrinsic sugars and a lower proportion from protein than those in non-benefit households.

Men and women in benefit households also:

- had lower mean daily intakes of non-starch polysaccharides compared with those in non-benefit households;
- tended to have lower vitamin intakes from food sources, although mean intakes for men and women were still above the RNI for all vitamins except vitamin A in women. Mean vitamin A intakes for women in benefit households were close to the RNI when intakes from supplements were included;

- had lower mean intakes of almost all minerals compared with those in non-benefit households. For example, mean daily intakes of magnesium for men were well below the RNI for those in benefit households but above the RNI for those in non-benefit households.
- A significantly higher proportion of women in benefit households had low intakes, that is below the LRNI, from food sources, of vitamin A and riboflavin compared with those in non-benefit households.
- A higher proportion of women living in benefit households had low intakes of all minerals from food sources compared with women in non-benefit households. For men, this was true for intakes of magnesium and potassium.

Figure 3.17 shows the proportion of respondents with intakes of iron below the LRNI by sex and household benefit status.

- More than half, 53%, of women aged 19 to 50 years living in benefit households had an iron intake from food sources below the LRNI, compared with about a third, 29%, of those in non-benefit households.

(Figure 3.17)

3.6 Comparison with 1986/87 Adults Survey

Table 3.9 compares total energy, macronutrient, vitamin and mineral intakes in the current survey of adults with corresponding data from the 1986/87 Adults Survey[2]. Comparisons are made between comparable age groups in the two surveys. It should be noted that in the 1986/87 Adults Survey the youngest age group was adults aged 16 to 24 years, while in the current NDNS the youngest age group is adults aged 19 to 24 years. This should be borne in mind where there are differences between these groups. A summary of the methodology and findings from the 1986/87 Adults Survey is given in Appendix S of the Technical Report[21].

Figure 3.18 shows the macronutrient composition of the diet for the 1986/87 Adults Survey and the 2000/01 NDNS.

- Men in the current survey had lower energy intakes compared with men in the 1986/87 Adults Survey.

Figure 3.17

Proportion of respondents with average daily intakes of iron (from food sources, that is excluding dietary supplements) below the Lower Reference Nutrient Intake (LRNI)* by sex of respondent and household benefit status

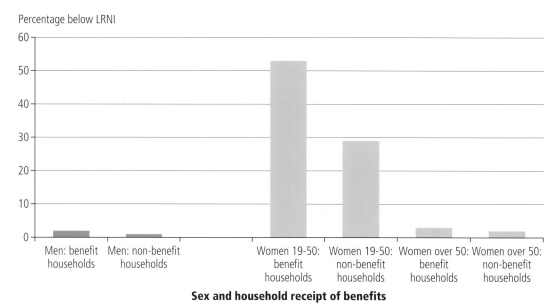

Percentage below LRNI

Sex and household receipt of benefits

* LRNIs for iron are set at 4.7mg/d for men, 8.0mg/d for women aged 19 to 50 years and 4.7mg/d for women over the age of 50.

- Men and women in the current survey derived more of their energy from protein and carbohydrate, and less from total fat and saturated fatty acids, than those in the 1986/87 Adults Survey.
- Mean intakes of total carbohydrate and total fat as a percentage of energy are currently close to recommended levels. Average intakes of saturated fatty acids as a percentage of energy have fallen, but remain well in excess of recommendations.
- Women in the 2000/01 NDNS obtained more of their energy from alcohol than those in the 1986/87 Adults Survey.

Changes in the macronutrient composition of the diet between the two surveys are in line with trends seen in the National Food Survey[22].

Mean daily intakes of vitamins and minerals are compared for intakes from food sources only, apart from magnesium, potassium and zinc where data from the 1986/87 Adults Survey is only available for intakes from all sources, including dietary supplements. More detailed information comparing intakes between the two surveys can be found in Volumes 2 and 3[4,5].

Compared with the 1986/87 Adults Survey, men and women in the current survey had:

Higher intakes of:
- folate;
- vitamin C;
- calcium;
- potassium; and
- vitamin D (women only).

The increase in intakes of vitamin D for women seen in the current survey is likely to be attributable in part to the revision of vitamin D values in poultry and meat and products[23].

Lower intakes of:
- vitamin A;
- copper; and
- zinc.

This fall in assessed intakes of vitamin A is largely due to revised data for retinol levels in liver and milk becoming available since the 1986/87 Adults Survey.

The extent to which these differences reflect changes in the diets of adults over the period is not clear. Many factors contribute to observed differences, including changes in nutrient composition, new analytical methods[23], increase in fortification practices, changes in food consumption patterns and increased use of dietary supplements.

Table 3.9

Comparison of average daily energy and micronutrient intakes and percentage contribution to energy intakes from macronutrients with the 1986/87 Adults Survey

Nutrients	Age of respondent (years)					Age of respondent (years)				
	1986/87 Adults Survey				All	2000/01 NDNS				All
	16–24	25–34	35–49	50–64	16–24	19–24	25–34	35–49	50–64	19–24
Men										
Mean daily total energy intake (MJ)	10.29	10.21	10.46	9.96	10.30	9.44	9.82	9.93	9.55	9.72
Protein										
% food energy from protein**	..	..	..	..	15.2	14.9	16.5	16.7	17.0	16.5
% total energy from protein	13.7	14.1	13.9	14.7	14.1	14.0	15.4	15.5	15.9	15.4
Total carbohydrate										
% food energy from carbohydrate**	..	..	..	..	44.7	49.0	47.7	47.5	47.4	47.7
% total energy from carbohydrate	42.9	40.9	41.5	41.4	41.6	46.0	44.6	44.4	44.6	44.7
Total fat										
% food energy from total fat	40.2	41.0	40.2	40.2	40.4	36.0	35.8	35.9	35.6	35.8
% total energy from total fat	37.9	37.9	37.1	37.6	37.6	34.0	33.5	33.4	33.3	33.5
Saturated fatty acids										
% food energy from saturated fatty acids	16.1	16.5	16.3	17.2	16.5	13.5	13.2	13.5	13.4	13.4
% total energy from saturated fatty acids	15.2	15.3	15.1	16.1	15.4	12.8	12.3	12.6	12.6	12.6
Alcohol***										
% total energy from alcohol	5.9	7.3	7.6	6.4	6.9	6.0	6.6	6.8	6.4	6.5
Mean daily intakes from food sources:										
Vitamin A (retinol equivalents) (µg)	1164	1552	1759	1897	1628	560	724	989	1145	911
Folate (µg)	302	317	321	300	311	301	346	343	361	344
Vitamin C (mg)	64.9	69.7	65.0	66.5	66.5	64.9	74.1	88.4	94.5	83.4
Vitamin D (µg)	2.8	3.2	3.7	3.8	3.4	2.9	3.5	3.7	4.2	3.7
Total iron (mg)	12.6	13.8	14.2	13.9	13.7	11.4	13.0	13.7	13.6	13.2
Calcium (mg)	894	931	960	949	937	860	1017	1040	1027	1007
Magnesium (mg)****	304	325	336	317	323	260	311	322	320	311
Potassium (mg)****	3018	3237	3279	3155	3187	2847	3286	3485	3553	3371
Zinc (mg)****	10.7	11.3	11.7	11.5	11.4	9.2	10.7	11.4	10.8	10.7
Copper (mg)	1.40	1.56	1.68	1.63	1.59	1.14	1.37	1.53	1.51	1.43
Base - number of men	*214*	*254*	*346*	*273*	*1087*	*108*	*219*	*253*	*253*	*833*

Nutrients	Age of respondent (years)				All	Age of respondent (years)				All
	1986/87 Adults Survey					2000/01 NDNS				
	16–24	25–34	35–49	50–64	16–24	19–24	25–34	35–49	50–64	19–24
Women										
Mean daily total energy intake (MJ)	7.11	6.99	7.24	6.74	7.05	7.00	6.61	6.96	6.91	6.87
Protein										
% food energy from protein**	..	..	..	..	15.6	15.4	15.9	16.7	17.4	16.6
% total energy from protein	14.0	14.6	15.4	16.1	15.2	14.8	15.3	16.1	16.8	15.9
Total carbohydrate										
% food energy from carbohydrate**	..	..	..	..	44.2	49.1	48.7	48.6	48.1	48.5
% total energy from carbohydrate	44.9	43.0	42.5	42.3	43.0	47.0	46.8	46.8	46.4	46.7
Total fat										
% food energy from total fat	39.8	40.7	40.3	40.3	40.3	35.5	35.4	34.7	34.5	34.9
% total energy from total fat	38.7	39.4	39.0	39.5	39.2	33.8	34.0	33.3	33.3	33.5
Saturated fatty acids										
% food energy from saturated fatty acids	16.4	16.9	16.9	17.5	17.0	12.9	13.2	13.2	13.3	13.2
% total energy from saturated fatty acids	16.0	16.4	16.4	17.1	16.5	12.8	12.3	12.6	12.6	12.6
Alcohol***										
% total energy from alcohol	2.5	3.1	3.2	2.2	2.8	4.6	4.0	3.9	3.7	3.9
Mean daily intakes from food sources:										
Vitamin A (retinol equivalents) (µg)	1051	1234	1531	1655	1413	467	587	675	816	671
Folate (µg)	198	206	220	218	213	229	234	255	268	251
Vitamin C (mg)	60.4	55.9	62.7	67.6	62.0	67.9	72.3	80.0	94.4	81.0
Vitamin D (µg)	2.1	2.3	2.6	2.8	2.5	2.3	2.4	2.8	3.5	2.8
Total iron (mg)	9.8	10.2	11.0	10.6	10.5	8.8	9.2	10.2	10.9	10.0
Calcium (mg)	675	699	760	739	726	694	731	796	823	777
Magnesium (mg)****	215	232	250	238	237	208	211	241	252	233
Potassium (mg)****	2259	2324	2562	2476	2434	2364	2398	2734	2885	2655
Zinc (mg)****	7.6	8.2	8.7	8.6	8.4	7.1	7.1	8.2	8.6	7.9
Copper (mg)	1.09	1.15	1.31	1.28	1.23	0.91	1.00	1.05	1.07	1.03
Base - number of women	189	253	385	283	1110	104	210	318	259	891

*   *1986/87 Gregory JR et al. The Dietary and Nutritional Survey of British Adults. HMSO (London, 1990).*

**   *Data on the percentage of food energy derived from protein and total carbohydrate are not available for the 1986/87 Adults Survey.*

*** *Data on the percentage of total energy derived from alcohol is based on the total sample, that is including non-consumers.*

**** *Data on intakes of these minerals are only available for all sources for 1986/87 Adults Survey. Data were not presented separately for intakes from food sources alone as dietary supplements only made a small contribution to intakes of these minerals.*

Figure 3.18(a)

Percentage contribution of macronutrients to average daily total energy intake: all men 1986/87 Adults Survey

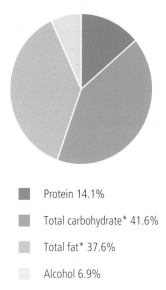

■	Protein 14.1%
■	Total carbohydrate* 41.6%
■	Total fat* 37.6%
■	Alcohol 6.9%

Figure 3.18(b)

Percentage contribution of macronutrients to average daily total energy intake: all men 2000/01 NDNS

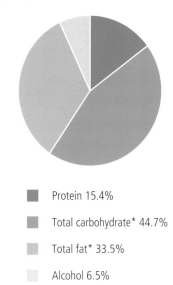

■	Protein 15.4%
■	Total carbohydrate* 44.7%
■	Total fat* 33.5%
■	Alcohol 6.5%

Figure 3.18(c)

Percentage contribution of macronutrients to average daily total energy intake: all women 1986/87 Adults Survey

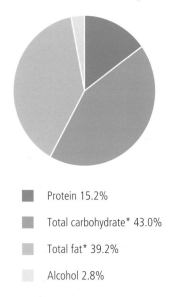

■	Protein 15.2%
■	Total carbohydrate* 43.0%
■	Total fat* 39.2%
■	Alcohol 2.8%

Figure 3.18(d)

Percentage contribution of macronutrients to average daily total energy intake: all women 2000/01 NDNS

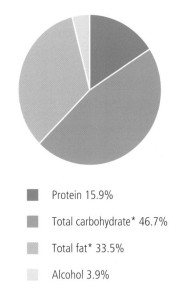

■	Protein 15.9%
■	Total carbohydrate* 46.7%
■	Total fat* 33.5%
■	Alcohol 3.9%

* DRVs for total carbohydrate and total fat are that the population average intake of total carbohydrate should not exceed 47% of total energy intake, and the population average intake of total fat should not exceed 33% of total energy intake.

3.7 Summary

Energy and macronutrient intakes (protein, total carbohydrate, non-milk extrinsic sugars, non-starch polysaccharides, total fat and saturated fatty acids):

- mean daily total energy intakes were below EARs for each sex and age group;
- mean percentage of food energy derived from total carbohydrate was near the DRV for all sex and age groups;
- mean percentage of food energy derived from non-milk extrinsic sugars was above the DRV for all sex and age groups except for the oldest group of women;
- mean daily intake of non-starch polysaccharides was below the recommended average intake of 18g per day for all sex and age groups;
- mean percentage of food energy derived from total fat was close to the DRV for each sex and age group; and
- mean percentage of food energy derived from saturated fatty acids was above the DRV for each sex and age group.

Alcohol consumption

- 60% of men and 44% of women exceeded the recommendations for alcohol consumption on at least 1 day during the seven-day dietary recording period (data not shown).
- Over a third of men, 39%, and over a fifth of women, 22%, drank heavily on at least one day during the survey week.
- Men aged 35 to 49 years were more likely to exceed the recommendation for alcohol consumption compared with the oldest group of men, and the youngest group of women compared with the oldest group of women.

Vitamin and mineral intakes

- Mean intakes of all vitamins from food sources were close to or above the RNI for all sex and age groups, except for vitamin A in the youngest group of men and women.
- Mean intakes of some minerals (e.g. iron, magnesium, potassium and copper) were well below the RNI for a number of sex and age groups.
- There was evidence of low intakes of vitamin A, riboflavin, magnesium and potassium for men and women, particularly in the youngest age groups, and of iodine in the youngest group of women.

- Over 40% of the two youngest groups of women had low intakes of iron.
- Dietary supplements had little effect on the number of people with low intakes.

Salt intakes

- Mean intakes of salt exceeded the 6g per day recommendation in all sex and age groups, and were higher for men (11.0g) than for women (8.1g).
- 15% of men and 31% of women had salt intakes of 6g per day or less, on average, over the survey week.
- Mean salt intakes for men and women have increased slightly from 9g per day in 1986/87 to 9.5g per day in 2000/01.

Differences in nutrient intakes by region

- There were few clear regional differences in intakes of energy, macronutrients or vitamins and minerals for men or women.

Differences in nutrient intakes by household receipt of benefits

- Adults living in households in receipt of benefits had lower average intakes of energy and some nutrients, particularly vitamins and minerals, compared with adults in non-benefit households.
- A higher proportion of women in benefit households had low intakes of vitamin A, riboflavin, folate and all minerals than those in non-benefit households.

Comparison with the 1986/87 Adults Survey

- Men in the current survey had lower total energy intakes than men in the 1986/87 Adults Survey.
- Men and women in the current survey derived more of their energy from protein and carbohydrate, and less from total fat and saturated fatty acids, than those in the 1986/87 Adults Survey.
- Women in the 2000/01 NDNS obtained more of their energy from alcohol than those in the 1986/87 Adults Survey.
- Men and women in the current survey had higher intakes of folate, vitamin C, calcium, potassium and, for women only, of vitamin D, and lower intakes of vitamin A, copper and zinc than those in the 1986/87 Adults Survey.

References and endnotes

[1] Mis-reporting (usually under-reporting) of foods consumed is a well recognised and unavoidable problem in dietary surveys. It was not possible to correct the data for this. However, the best dietary methodology was used which aimed to minimise mis-reporting. In addition, fieldworkers who collect the dietary information are trained to check the dietary records and remind people about foods that are commonly forgotten.

[2] Gregory J, Foster K, Tyler H, Wiseman M. *The Dietary and Nutritional Survey of British Adults.* HMSO (London, 1990).

[3] Nutrients not presented in this volume are: intrinsic and milk sugars, starch, *trans* fatty acids, *cis* monounsaturated fatty acids, *cis* n-3 polyunsaturated fatty acids, *cis* n-6 polyunsaturated fatty acids, cholesterol, pre-formed retinol, total carotene, ∝-carotene, β-carotene, β-cryptoxanthin, biotin, pantothenic acid, vitamin E, haem iron, non-haem iron, phosphorus, and manganese. Information on intakes and food sources of these nutrients can be found in Volumes 2 and 3 (*see* Notes 4 and 5).

[4] Henderson L, Gregory J, Irving K, Swan G. *National Diet and Nutrition Survey: adults aged 19 to 64 years. Volume 2: Energy, protein, carbohydrate, fat and alcohol intake.* TSO (London, 2003).

[5] Henderson L, Irving K, Gregory J, Bates CJ, Prentice A, Perks J, Swan G, Farron M. *National Diet and Nutrition Survey: adults aged 19 to 64 years. Volume 3: Vitamin and mineral intake and urinary analytes.* TSO (London, 2003).

[6] Department of Health. Report on Health and Social Subjects: **41**. *Dietary Reference Values for Food Energy and Nutrients for the United Kingdom.* HMSO (London, 1991).

[7] Department of Health. *Dietary Reference Values. A Guide.* HMSO (London, 1991).

[8] Alcohol Concern. *Factsheet 8: Health impacts of alcohol.* **35**. Winter 2002/03.

[9] Department of Health. *Sensible drinking - the report of an inter-departmental working group.* HMSO (London, 1996).

[10] Data from the dietary interview can be used to calculate weekly consumption of alcohol in units. However, as the revised guidelines focus on maximum daily consumption we cannot simply divide weekly consumption by seven as this would give average daily consumption. It was decided, therefore, to use the information collected in the dietary record to estimate maximum daily units consumed.

[11] Department of Health. Report on health and social subjects: **50**. *Folic acid and the preventionof disease: report of the Committee on Medical Aspects of Food and Nutrition Policy.* TSO (London, 2000).

[12] Intakes as a percentage of the RNI were calculated for each respondent, taking the appropriate RNI for each sex/age group. The values for all respondents in each age group were then pooled to give a mean value.

[13] Hard water typically provides 200mg calcium daily, while in soft water areas it provides none. Due to regional differences it was not possible to ascertain the contribution of water to calcium intake. In addition, it was not possible to distinguish whether tap water consumed had been filtered, which would reduce, for example, the levels of calcium, chloride and heavy metals found in tap water.

[14] Department of Health. Report on Health and Social Subjects: **46**. *Nutritional Aspects of Cardiovascular Disease.* HMSO (London, 1994).

[15] Scientific Advisory Committee on Nutrition. *Salt and Health.* TSO (London, 2003). The Scientific Advisory Committee on Nutrition found no basis for a revision of the 1994 COMA recommendation for a target salt intake of 6g/day (2.4g/100mmol sodium) for the adult population. Six grams is higher than the Reference Nutrient Intake (RNI) and substantially greater than the salt intake required to maintain the sodium content of the body.

[16] Urine samples from respondents who reported making a complete 24 hour urine collection were tested for sodium levels. The results were then used to estimate salt intakes. For further information *see* Volume 3 (Note 5) and the Technical Report (Note 21).

[17] Includes the use of a salt alternative in cooking.

[18] Excludes the use of salt added in cooking or at the table.

[19] The areas included in each of the four analysis 'regions' are given in the response chapter, Chapter 2 of the Technical Report (*see* Note 21). Definitions of 'regions' are given in the glossary (*see* Appendix F).

[20] Households receiving benefits are those where someone in the respondent's household was currently receiving Working Families Tax Credit or had, in the previous 14 days, drawn Income Support or (Income-related) Job Seeker's Allowance. Definitions of 'household' and 'benefits (receiving)' are given in the glossary (*see* Appendix F).

[21] The Technical Report is available online at http://www.food.gov.uk/science.

[22] Department for Environment, Food & Rural Affairs. *National Food Survey 2000.* TSO (London, 2001). The National Food Survey was replaced by the Expenditure and Food Survey from 1 April 2001.

[23] Measurable amounts of vitamin D and its metabolites have now been found in meats as a result of new analytical methods.

4 Nutritional status (physical measurements and blood analytes), blood pressure and physical activity

4.1 Introduction

Nutritional status is a general term which provides an indication of how well-nourished an individual or group of people are. This includes the assessment of the levels and functional adequacy of nutrients available to the body after absorption for use in metabolic processes. Whereas nutrient intakes are estimated from food consumption over a short period (seven days in this survey), many measures of nutritional status indicate long term body stores. Poor nutritional status does not necessarily indicate clinical deficiency. There is a difference between the amount of a nutrient required to prevent clinical deficiency, for example, vitamin C and scurvy, and the amount required to achieve optimal status for a given nutrient.

Nutritional status is described here by reporting physical measurements (body mass index, waist circumference and waist to hip ratio) and results of the blood sample analyses. Blood samples were obtained with the respondents' consent and analysed for a range of components indicative of nutritional status, such as serum ferritin, which gives an indication of the level of iron stores in the body. This chapter also discusses the blood pressure measurements and physical activity, derived from information recorded in the physical activity diary. Where appropriate, results are compared against reference values or current recommendations. In addition, for physical measurements, data from the Dietary and Nutritional Survey of British Adults aged 16 to 64 years carried out in 1986/87 (1986/87 Adults Survey)[1] are presented for comparison. The response rate for each measurement is given in Appendix B. For full details on how the survey was weighted for each of these components, *see* Appendix B.

More specifically this chapter looks at:

- Physical measurements
  - body mass index;
  - waist circumference; and
  - waist to hip ratio

- Blood pressure

- Blood sample analysis
  - iron status;
  - status of vitamins A, B_1 (thiamin), B_2 (riboflavin), B_6, B_{12}, C, D, E and folate; and
  - cholesterol

- Physical activity

Detailed information on the protocols for taking these measurements is available in the Technical Report[2]. More detailed findings in relation to these measures, and other indices, including height and weight measurements, and additional blood sample analyses, can be found in Volume 4[3].

4.2 Physical measurements

4.2.1 Body mass index

Being overweight or obese increases the risk of heart disease, Type 2 diabetes, high blood pressure and osteoarthritis. When someone is obese, it means they are overweight to the point that it could seriously endanger their health[4].

Body weight alone is not a good indicator of obesity, or a useful predictor of health status as it is strongly correlated with height. However, weight can be adjusted for height to give an indicator of body shape that is independent of height and provides a measure of 'fatness'.

The most widely used measure of 'fatness' is the Quetelet or Body Mass Index (BMI). BMI is calculated as weight (kg) / height (m2) and in adults is customarily grouped as follows[5]:

Descriptor	BMI Index
Underweight	18.5 or less
Desirable	over 18.5 to 25
Overweight	over 25 to 30
Obese	over 30

There is a disadvantage to using BMI, however, because it may give potentially misleading levels of 'fatness' in lean individuals with muscular physiques since it is solely based on measurements of height and weight. However, BMI remains the most pragmatic and appropriate measure to assess obesity on a population basis. It is also recognised that the health risks of obesity are compounded when fat is distributed around the middle of the body. Thus another useful measurement is waist circumference, or waist to hip ratio (*see* Sections 4.2.2 and 4.2.3). Therefore someone who is overweight and has a high waist to hip ratio will be at greater risk of obesity related illness.

Table 4.1 shows the percentage distribution of BMI according to the above classification by sex and age. Figures 4.1(a) and (b) show distribution of BMI for men and women respectively.

- 25% of men and 20% of women were obese, and a further 42% of men and 32% of women were overweight.
- Men were more likely to be overweight or obese than women (that is, BMI over 25).
- For both men and women, older adults were more likely to be overweight than younger adults:
  - men in the two oldest age groups were more likely to be classified as overweight than those in the youngest age group, and those in the oldest group were more likely to be classified as obese than those aged 25 to 34 years; and
  - women aged 50 to 64 years were more likely to be classified as overweight than those in any other age group.
- 1% of men and 3% of women, overall, were classified as underweight. The proportion classified as underweight was highest for the youngest group of women, where 7% had a BMI of 18.5 or less.

(Table 4.1)
(Figures 4.1(a) and (b))

Table 4.2 compares data from the current survey with BMI measurements from the 1986/87 Adults Survey[1]. Comparisons are made between comparable age groups in the two surveys. It should be noted that in the 1986/87 Adults Survey the youngest age group was aged 16 to 24 years, while in the current NDNS the youngest age group was adults aged 19 to 24 years. This should be remembered where there are differences between these groups. Comparisons have only been made between adults classified as overweight or obese in

both surveys, as the classifications for underweight and desirable have been amended since the 1986/87 Adults Survey. A summary of the methodology and findings from the 1986/87 Adults Survey is given in Appendix S of the Technical Report[2].

Compared with the 1986/87 Adults Survey:

- a higher proportion of men and women in this survey were classified as overweight or obese (that is, BMI over 25). 66% of men and 53% of women were overweight or obese in this survey, compared with 45% of men and 36% of women in the 1986/87 Adults survey; and
- a higher proportion of men and women were classified as obese, 25% of men and 20% of women were obese in this survey compared with 8% of men and 12% of women in the 1986/87 Adults survey.

By age:

- a higher proportion of women aged 25 to 34 years and 50 to 64 years were classified as overweight in this survey; and
- a higher proportion of men in all age groups, and of women aged 35 to 49 years, were classified as obese in this survey.

(Table 4.2)

4.2.2 Waist circumference

Waist circumference is used as a measure to show increased risk of metabolic complications of obesity, for example, resistance to insulin by the body.

Guidelines suggest that for men a waist circumference greater than 102cm, and for women greater than 88cm, indicates a substantially increased risk of metabolic complications of obesity[5].

Table 4.1

Percentage distribution of BMI by classification by sex and age of respondent

BMI (kg/m²)	Men aged (years):				All men	Women aged (years):				All women
	19–24	25–34	35–49	50–64		19–24	25–34	35–49	50–64	
	%	%	%	%	%	%	%	%	%	%
Underweight (18.5 or less)	7	1	0	-	1	7	4	1	3	3
Desirable (over 18.5 to 25)	50	38	30	22	32	55	52	46	33	45
Overweight (over 25 to 30)	25	42	45	46	42	25	28	31	41	32
Obese (over 30)	18	18	25	32	25	14	16	23	22	20
Base	*110*	*227*	*263*	*264*	*864*	*110*	*213*	*331*	*269*	*922*

Figure 4.1(a)

Percentage distribution of BMI by classification and sex of respondent: men

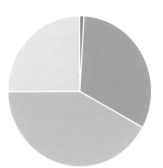

■ Underweight (18.5 or less) (1%)

■ Desirable (over 18.5 to 25) (32%)

■ Overweight (over 25 to 30) (42%)

■ Obese (over 30) (25%)

Figure 4.1(b)

Percentage distribution of BMI by classification and sex of respondent: women

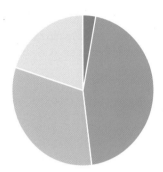

■ Underweight (18.5 or less) (3%)

■ Desirable (over 18.5 to 25) (45%)

■ Overweight (over 25 to 30) (32%)

■ Obese (over 30) (20%)

Data given below is taken from Volume 4[3].

- Overall, 29% of men had a waist circumference greater than 102cm and 26% of women had a waist circumference greater than 88cm.
- A higher proportion of the oldest group of men had a waist circumference greater than 102cm than men in any other age group.
- A higher proportion of women in the two oldest age groups had a waist circumference greater than 88cm than the youngest group of women.

4.2.3 Waist to hip ratio

The waist to hip ratio is a measure of the distribution of body fat (both subcutaneous and intra-abdominal). The ratio is calculated as waist circumference (cm) / hip circumference (cm) and is an indicator of the amount of fat deposited around the middle of the body. Guidelines suggest that for men a waist to hip ratio of 0.95 or greater, and for women 0.85 or greater, carries a potential health risk, for example, increased risk of cardio-vascular disease and diabetes[6].

Table 4.2

Comparison of distribution of BMI with the 1986/87 Adults Survey*

BMI (kg/m²)	Age of respondent (years):									
	1986/87 Adults Survey*				All	2000/01 NDNS				All
	16–24	25–34	35–49	50–64	16–64	19–24	25–34	35–49	50–64	19–64
	%	%	%	%	%	%	%	%	%	%
Men										
Overweight (over 25 to 30)	18	30	41	53	37	25	42	45	46	42
Obese (over 30)	3	6	11	9	8	18	18	25	32	25
Base	*222*	*269*	*369*	*298*	*1158*	*110*	*227*	*263*	*264*	*864*
Women										
Overweight (over 25 to 30)	17	16	30	28	24	24	28	31	41	32
Obese (over 30)	6	11	16	18	12	14	16	23	22	20
Base	*193*	*261*	*402*	*305*	*1161*	*110*	*213*	*331*	*269*	*922*

* *Gregory JR et al. The Dietary and Nutritional Survey of British Adults. HMSO (London, 1990).*

- Men had a greater mean waist to hip ratio, 0.90, than women, 0.79, and this was true for all age groups.
- 23% of men and 15 % of women had a waist to hip ratio that was above the guidelines.
- A higher proportion of the two oldest groups of men had a waist to hip ratio that was 0.95 or greater than men in the two youngest age groups.
- A higher proportion of women aged 50 to 64 years had a waist to hip ratio that was 0.85 or greater than women in any other age group.

For more details on waist to hip ratio, *see* Chapter 2 of Volume 4[3].

4.3 Blood pressure

Blood pressure is the term used to describe the opposing forces of blood pumped by the heart and the resistance of the blood vessels to flow. Systolic blood pressure is the peak pressure, which occurs when the heart contracts; diastolic blood pressure is the minimum pressure which occurs when the heart relaxes. Conventionally, blood pressure is presented as systolic blood pressure / diastolic blood pressure.

A higher than average blood pressure may lead to an increased risk of suffering heart disease or a stroke. A habitually higher intake of salt has been linked to a higher than average blood pressure. However, lifestyle factors, such as body weight, alcohol consumption and physical activity can also affect blood pressure. High blood pressure can also be hereditary.

The latest guidelines on the management of hypertension (high blood pressure) issued by the World Health Organization (WHO)[7] indicate that both hypertension and 'high normal' blood pressure pose a threat to health[8]. According to the guidelines, blood pressures are classified as follows.

- Hypertension: 140/90mmHg or above.
- High normal blood pressure: between 130/85mmHg and 140/90mmHg.
- Normal blood pressure: less than 130/85mmHg.
- Optimal blood pressure: less than 120/80mmHg.

For more discussion on the blood pressure measurements and guidelines, *see* Chapter 3 of Volume 4[3].

4.3.1 Systolic blood pressure

Table 4.3 shows the distribution of blood pressure according to the WHO guidelines[7], by sex and age.

Overall:

- 22% of men and 13% of women had systolic blood pressure that is considered hypertensive, and an additional 25% of men and 13% of women had systolic blood pressure that is considered 'high normal'.
- 24% of men and 51% of women had systolic blood pressure that is considered optimal.

By age

- Men and women in the oldest age group were more likely than those in any other age group to have systolic blood pressure that is classified as hypertensive. In addition, women aged 35 to 49 years were more likely than the youngest group to have systolic blood pressure that is classified as hypertensive.
- Men and women in the oldest age group were also less likely to have systolic blood pressure that is classified as optimal compared with those aged 25 to 34 years. This was also true for the oldest group of women compared with the youngest group.

4.3.2 Diastolic blood pressure

Table 4.3 also shows the distribution of diastolic blood pressure according to the WHO guidelines[7], and that:

- 7% of men and 3% of women had diastolic blood pressure that is considered hypertensive, that is at or above 90mmHg.
- 71% of men and 86% of women had diastolic blood pressure that is considered optimal.

By age

- Men in the two oldest age groups were more likely than those aged 25 to 34 years to have a diastolic blood pressure classified as hypertensive.
- Men and women in the youngest age group were more likely to have diastolic blood pressure classified as optimal than any other age group. For example, 100% of men and women aged 19 to 24 years had diastolic blood pressure classified as optimal, compared with 62% of men and 85% of women aged 35 to 49 years.

- In addition, men aged 25 to 34 years were more likely than those aged 35 to 64 years, and women aged 25 to 34 years were more likely than those aged 50 to 64 years to have diastolic blood pressure that is classified as optimal.

(Table 4.3)

4.4 Blood sample analysis

The following section presents results of the analysis of respondent blood samples. Table 4.4 describes the thresholds for each of the blood analytes considered, and Tables 4.5 to 4.8 show the percentage of respondents with levels outside these thresholds. For each analyte presented here a threshold level has been set to indicate the 'normal' range. Levels outside these thresholds indicate low status. Not all blood analytes are presented here[9]. For further information on these analytes, and details on additional analytes, *see* Chapter 4 of Volume 4[3].

4.4.1 Iron status

A number of indices of iron status were measured in the blood samples. This section focuses on three of these measures: haemoglobin concentration, percentage saturation of plasma iron and serum ferritin.

Haemoglobin concentration (grams/decilitre)

Haemoglobin is the oxygen-carrying, iron-containing molecule in red blood cells. Circulating levels of haemoglobin are indicative of the oxygen-carrying capacity of the blood. A low haemoglobin concentration can indicate iron deficiency. The WHO lower limits for haemoglobin concentration are 13.0g/dl for men and 12.0g/dl for women[10]. Concentrations lower than these are indicative of anaemia. The haemoglobin concentrations of women of childbearing age tend to be lower because of menstrual losses.

Table 4.5 shows that:

- 8% of women and 3% of men were anaemic, that is, they had low levels of haemoglobin in their blood (that is, a haemoglobin concentration below the WHO lower limit).

Percentage saturation of plasma iron (%)

Iron is bound to transferrin, a protein, for transportation around the body. A decrease in the percentage saturation of transferrin with iron is an indicator of a progressive iron deficiency state with depleted iron stores. When the percentage transferrin saturation drops to a certain level haemoglobin formation is likely to be impaired. For adults this level is usually considered to be 15%[11].

- Women were more likely than men to have low plasma iron percentage saturation, 16% compared with 7%.

Serum ferritin (micrograms/litre)

Serum ferritin gives an indication of the level of iron stores, where low concentrations are an indication of low iron stores in the body. The normal range for serum ferritin is generally taken to be 20µg/l to 300µg/l for men and 15µg/l to 150µg/l for women[12].

Table 4.3

Percentage distribution of blood pressure by classification and by sex and age of respondent

BP (mmHg)	Men aged (years):				All men	Women aged (years):				All women
	19–24	25–34	35–49	50–64		19–24	25–34	35–49	50–64	
	%	%	%	%	%	%	%	%	%	%
Systolic										
Optimal (less than 120)	28	33	24	16	24	74	69	52	24	51
Normal (120 and less than 130)	39	30	35	19	29	20	24	27	19	23
High normal (130 and less than 140)	22	24	23	28	25	5	4	14	24	13
Hypertension (140 and above)	12	14	18	37	22	1	3	7	33	13
Diastolic										
Optimal (less than 80)	100	88	62	55	71	100	91	85	76	86
Normal (80 and less than 85)	-	8	17	20	13	-	6	8	12	7
High normal (85 and less than 90)	-	2	12	13	8	-	1	5	6	4
Hypertension (90 and above)	-	2	9	12	7	-	2	3	6	3
Base	*109*	*221*	*255*	*255*	*839*	*105*	*212*	*320*	*260*	*897*

As shown in Table 4.5:

- 11% of women and 4% of men had low levels of serum ferritin.

(Tables 4.4 and 4.5)

4.4.2 Water soluble vitamins

Respondents' blood samples were tested for a range of analytes which reflect levels of the following water soluble vitamins in the body: vitamin C; folate; vitamin B_{12}; thiamin; riboflavin and vitamin B_6. Table 4.6 shows the proportion of respondents, by sex and age, with low levels of these water soluble vitamins.

Plasma vitamin C (micromoles/litre)

Vitamin C is needed for the maintenance of healthy connective tissue in the body, acts as an antioxidant protecting cells from the damage caused by free radicals, and helps in the absorption of iron. Plasma vitamin C concentrations reflect recent dietary intakes of vitamin C, with values of less than 11μmol/l indicative of biochemical depletion[13].

Table 4.6 shows that:

- 5% of men and 3% of women had a plasma vitamin C concentration below 11μmol/l.

Red cell folate and serum folate (nanomoles/litre)

The B vitamin folate is a general term for a group of compounds (folic acid and derivatives). Folate has several functions, including its action with vitamin B_{12} to form healthy red blood cells. *Red cell* folate is usually a better measure of long-term status than *plasma* folate because it reflects body stores at the time red blood cells are made. The folate status of women of childbearing age is a particular public health issue. Poor folate status in women of child-bearing age is linked to an increased risk of having babies with neural tube defects including spina bifida (*see* Chapter 3)[14].

In adults, a *red cell* folate concentration below 230nmol/l is considered to be severely deficient, while concentrations between 230nmol/l and 345nmol/l indicate marginal status[15]. The normal range for *serum* folate concentration in adults is usually considered to be between 7nmol/l and 46nmol/l, with concentrations less than 6.3nmol/l being considered deficient[12].

Table 4.6 shows that:

- 4% of men and 5% of women had a concentration of *red cell* folate indicating marginal status.
- No more than 1% of any sex/age group had a *red cell* folate concentration indicative of severe red cell folate deficiency.
- 1% of men and less than 0.5% of women had a *serum folate* concentration below the lower level of the normal range.
- 8% of the youngest group of women and 4% of those aged 25 to 34 years had a concentration of *red cell* folate indicating marginal status.

Serum vitamin B_{12} (picomoles/litre)

Vitamin B_{12}, with folate, is required for protein processing, DNA synthesis and to maintain the nervous system. Poor vitamin B_{12} status may be due to low dietary intake, poor absorption or pernicious anaemia. Serum concentration of vitamin B_{12} is a good indicator of vitamin B_{12} status. For adults, the lower level of normality for serum vitamin B_{12} concentration is usually taken as 118pmol/l[12].

- Overall, 2% of men and 4% of women had a serum vitamin B_{12} concentration below the limit of the normal range.

Vitamin B_1 (thiamin) – Erythrocyte Transketolase Activation Coefficient (ETKAC)

Thiamin has a number of important functions in the body. For example, it is necessary for the release and utilisation of energy from food and is required to ensure a healthy nervous system. Transketolase is a red cell enzyme that depends on a co-factor derived from thiamin. *The Erythrocyte Transketolase Activation Coefficient* (ETKAC) index measures the extent to which transketolase has been depleted of this co-factor – indicating the level of adequacy of thiamin in the body. The ETKAC is an index that is sensitive to the lower to moderate range of intakes of thiamin. For adults, values above 1.25 are indicative of biochemical thiamin deficiency[11].

Table 4.6 shows that:

- 3% of men and 1% of women had a mean ETKAC greater than 1.25.

Table 4.4

Blood analytes indicating the thresholds for status

Blood analyte (units)	Men	Women
Iron status		
Haemoglobin concentration (g/dl)		
lower threshold for anaemia	less than 13.0	less than 12.0
% Iron saturation* (%)		
lower threshold for anaemia	less than 15.0	less than 15.0
Serum ferritin (µg/l)		
low iron stores	less than 20	less than 15
Water soluble vitamins		
Plasma vitamin C (µmol/l)		
biochemical depletion	less than 11	less than 11
Red cell folate (nmol/l)**		
severely deficient	less than 230	less than 230
marginal status	230 to less than 345	230 to less than 345
Serum folate (nmol/l)		
deficient	less than 6.3	less than 6.3
Serum vitamin B_{12} (pmol/l)		
lower limit of normal range	less than 118	less than 118
Thiamin (ETKAC) (ratio)		
biochemical thiamin deficiency	above 1.25	above 1.25
Riboflavin (EGRAC) (ratio)		
marginal/deficient status	above 1.3	above 1.3
Vitamin B_6 (EAATAC) (ratio)		
biochemical vitamin B_6 deficiency	above 2.0	above 2.0
Fat soluble vitamins		
Plasma retinol (µmol/l)		
severely deficient	less than 0.35	less than 0.35
marginal status	0.35 to less than 0.70	0.35 to less than 0.70
Plasma 25-hydroxyvitamin D (nmol/l)		
lower limit of normal range	less than 25	less than 25
Tocopherol: cholesterol ratio (µmol/mmol)***		
lower limit of normal range	less than 2.25	less than 2.25
Blood lipids		
Plasma total cholesterol (mmol/l)		
optimal level	less than 5.2	less than 5.2
mildly elevated	5.2 to 6.4	5.2 to 6.4
moderately elevated	6.5 to 7.8	6.5 to 7.8
severely elevated	higher than 7.8	higher than 7.8

*   *Measured as percentage saturation of total iron-binding capacity in plasma.*

**   *Concentrations of red cell folate between 230 and 345nmol/l represent marginal status. To maintain consistency across volumes, data outside these ranges are reported as in Chapter 4, Volume 4 (ie % between 230 and 350 not 345nmol/l).*

*** *∝-tocopherol to total cholesterol ratio.*

Table 4.5

Percentage of respondents below thresholds for iron status including haemoglobin, by sex and age of respondent

Blood analyte	Men aged (years):				All men	Women aged (years):				All women
	19–24	25–34	35–49	50–64		19–24	25–34	35–49	50–64	
	%	%	%	%	%	%	%	%	%	%
Haemoglobin concentration										
lower threshold for anaemia	-	2	4	3	3	7	8	10	7	8
% Iron saturation										
lower threshold for anaemia	6	13	3	6	7	27	17	18	8	16
Serum ferritin										
low iron stores	4	0	6	5	4	16	8	12	8	11

Vitamin B$_2$ (riboflavin) – Erythrocyte Glutathione Reductase Activation Coefficient (EGRAC)

Riboflavin has many functions, including being needed for the utilisation of energy from food. The *Erythrocyte Glutathione Reductase Activation Coefficient* (EGRAC) is a measure of red cell enzyme saturation with its riboflavin-derived-cofactor, flavin adenine dinucleotide. It should be noted that the EGRAC index is very sensitive and detects small degrees of riboflavin depletion in the tissues, leading to a high proportion of raised values indicating poor status. The significance of these slightly raised values for health is unclear. A coefficient of between 1.0 and 1.3 is generally considered to be normal. Levels above 1.3 indicate poor status.

- Two-thirds of men and women had a mean EGRAC greater than 1.3.
- Men in the youngest age group, and women aged 19 to 49 years, were more likely than those in the oldest age group to have an EGRAC greater than 1.3.

Vitamin B$_6$ – Erythrocyte Aspartate Aminotransferase Activation Coefficient (EAATAC)

The *Erythrocyte Aspartate Aminotransferase Activation Coefficient* (EAATAC) is a measure of the saturation of a red cell enzyme with a co-factor derived from vitamin B$_6$. For adults, values above 2.00 are indicative of biochemical vitamin B$_6$ deficiency[12].

- Overall, 10% of men and 11% of women had an EAATAC greater than 2.00, suggesting biochemical vitamin B$_6$ deficiency.

(Tables 4.4 and 4.6)

4.4.3 Fat soluble vitamins

Respondents' blood samples were tested for a range of analytes which reflect levels of the following fat soluble vitamins in the body: vitamin A; vitamin D and vitamin E. Table 4.7 shows the proportion of respondents, by sex and age, with low levels of these fat soluble vitamins.

Plasma retinol (vitamin A) (micromoles/litre)

Vitamin A is essential for maintaining and repairing tissues needed for growth and normal development. It also helps to maintain healthy skin and mucus linings such as in the nose. Vitamin A also helps strengthen immunity from infections and is essential for vision in dim light. Although plasma retinol is related to long-term dietary intake of vitamin A, the strongest associations are only when intake is low or high. At normal levels of intake, the plasma concentration is naturally controlled in the body with little variation either within or between subjects. For adults, concentrations below 0.35µmol/l are considered to be severely deficient and concentrations between 0.35µmol/l and 0.70µmol/l indicate marginal status[11].

Table 4.7 shows that:

- None of the respondents who provided a blood sample, had plasma retinol values indicating severe vitamin A deficiency.
- 1% of men aged 50 to 64 years had plasma retinol concentrations indicating marginal status. No other age groups for men or any groups for women had marginal status for plasma retinol concentrations.

Table 4.6

Percentage of respondents with poor status for water soluble vitamins by sex and age of respondent

Blood analyte	Men aged (years):				All men	Women aged (years):				All women
	19–24	25–34	35–49	50–64		19–24	25–34	35–49	50–64	
	%	%	%	%	%	%	%	%	%	%
Plasma vitamin C										
biochemical depletion	7	5	4	5	5	4	3	4	3	3
Red cell folate										
severely deficient	-	1	1	-	1	-	-	-	0	0
marginal status*	13	3	4	2	4	8	4	5	6	5
Serum folate										
deficient	-	1	1	1	1	-	-	0	-	0
Serum vitamin B$_{12}$										
below lower limit of normal range	-	-	2	3	2	5	5	4	3	4
Thiamin (ETKAC)**										
biochemical thiamin deficiency	-	3	2	5	3	-	1	2	1	1
Riboflavin (EGRAC)**										
marginal/deficient status	82	70	67	54	66	77	78	69	50	66
Vitamin B$_6$ (EAATAC)**										
biochemical vitamin B$_6$ deficiency	4	10	13	11	10	12	8	12	13	11

*   Data presented are for red cell folate greater than 230nmol/l and less than 350nmol/l as in Chapter 4, Volume 4, not 345nmol/l as quoted in Table 4.4.

** Values above the threshold indicate low status.

Plasma 25-hydroxyvitamin D (nanomoles/litre)

Plasma 25-hydroxyvitamin D (25-OHD) is a measure of vitamin D status and reflects the availability of vitamin D in the body. Vitamin D is required for calcium absorption as well as for a range of other metabolic processes. Vitamin D is obtained both through the action of sunlight on the skin and from the diet. Therefore, factors related to sunlight exposure, such as the time of year, habit of dress and time spent outdoors should be considered when interpreting these results. Traditionally 25nmol/l has been used as the lower threshold for plasma 25-OHD[16]. Table 4.7 and Figure 4.2 show the proportion of respondents below this threshold by sex and age.

- Overall, 14% of men and 15% of women had a plasma 25-OHD concentration lower than 25nmol/l. The proportion of men and women in the youngest age group with a plasma 25-OHD concentration below the threshold was higher, 24% and 28% respectively.

(Table 4.7 and Figure 4.2)

Seasonal variation in concentration of plasma 25-OHD

Plasma concentrations of 25-OHD are likely to be higher during the summer months as vitamin D made through the action of sunlight on the skin is an important source. Figure 4.3 shows the seasonal variation in the proportion of respondents below the vitamin D threshold by sex and age.

- Men who provided a sample of blood during July to September were significantly less likely to have a 25-OHD concentration below 25nmol/l than those who gave a sample at other times of the year.
- Women providing a sample of blood in July to September were significantly less likely to have a 25-OHD concentration below 25nmol/l compared with those providing a sample in January to March or April to June.
- Nearly one quarter of men and women who provided a sample in the months January to March had a 25-OHD concentration below 25nmol/l.

(Figure 4.3)

Table 4.7

Percentage of respondents with poor status for fat soluble vitamins by sex and age of respondent

Blood analyte	Men aged (years):				All men	Women aged (years):				All women
	19–24	25–34	35–49	50–64		19–24	25–34	35–49	50–64	
	%	%	%	%	%	%	%	%	%	%
Plasma retinol										
severely deficient	-	-	-	-	-	-	-	-	-	-
marginal status	-	-	-	1	0	-	-	-	-	-
Plasma 25-hydroxyvitamin D										
below lower limit of normal range	24	16	12	9	14	28	13	15	11	15
Tocopherol: cholesterol ratio*										
below lower limit of normal range	1	1	1	1	1	-	2	1	3	2

* ∝-tocopherol to total cholesterol ratio.

Tocopherol to cholesterol ratio (vitamin E) (micromoles/millimoles)

Vitamin E has an important role in the body as an antioxidant, protecting cells from the damage caused by free radicals. Plasma tocopherol can be used as a measure of vitamin E status. Plasma tocopherol can be usefully expressed as a ratio of tocopherol to cholesterol (µmol/mmol)[17], enabling comparisons to be made between age groups with different plasma lipid levels. For adults, a tocopherol to cholesterol ratio of below 2.25µmol/mmol is considered to be the lowest satisfactory value[18].

- 1% of men and 2% of women had a tocopherol to cholesterol ratio below 2.25µmol/mmol.

(Tables 4.4 and 4.7)

4.4.4 Blood lipids

Plasma cholesterol (millimoles/litre)

In adults, circulating levels of plasma total cholesterol and its subfractions (for example LDL and HDL cholesterol) are among the predictors of coronary heart disease (CHD)[19]. Levels vary with age, genetic and environmental influences, including dietary factors, notably the amount of saturated fatty acids in the diet. The absolute risk of CHD increases with age but the interactions of risk factors, including plasma cholesterol, cigarette smoking, high blood pressure and body weight obscure individual relationships with CHD. High levels of total cholesterol occur in some diseases, for example kidney, liver and thyroid disorders or in diabetes[20].

Figure 4.2

Proportion of respondents with low vitamin D status (less than 25nmol/l) by sex and age of respondent

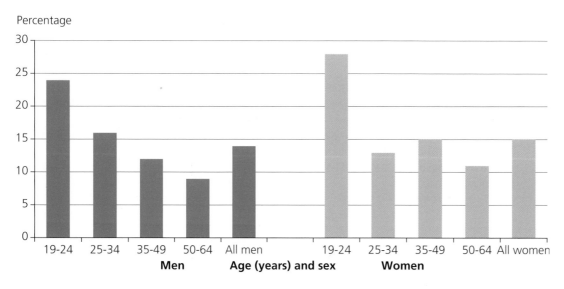

It is generally accepted that a plasma total cholesterol concentration below 5.2mmol/l represents an optimal level, 5.2mmol/l to 6.4mmol/l mildly elevated, 6.5mmol/l to 7.8mmol/l moderately elevated and above 7.8mmol/l a severely elevated level[20,21].

Table 4.8 shows that:

- Over half, 52%, of men and women had optimal plasma total cholesterol concentrations (that is, below 5.2mmol/l).
- The proportion with optimal plasma total cholesterol concentrations decreased with age for both men and women.
- Over a third of men and women had mildly elevated concentrations (that is, between 5.2mmol/l and 6.5mmol/l).
- 12% of men and 10% of women had moderately elevated cholesterol concentrations (that is, between 6.5mmol/l to 7.8mmol/l).
- 2% of men and 3% of women had severely elevated plasma total cholesterol concentrations (that is, 7.8mmol/l or above).
- None of the men or women aged 19 to 24 years had a moderately or severely elevated plasma total cholesterol concentration, that is, a mean concentration of 6.5mmol/l or above. The proportion of women with severely elevated levels increased from 1% of those aged 25 to 34 years to 9% of those aged 50 to 64 years.

4.5 Physical activity

The Health Development Agency and Health Survey for England give the following definitions of physical activity and exercise[22,23].

Physical activity

Any force exerted by skeletal muscle that results in energy expenditure above resting level.

Exercise

A subset of physical activity, which is volitional, planned, structured, repetitive and aimed at improvement or maintenance of any aspect of fitness or health.

Moderate intensity physical activity

Activities with an energy cost of at least 5 kcal/min but less than 7.5 kcal/min, usually equivalent to brisk walking, which might be expected to leave the participant feeling warm or slightly out of breath.

Vigorous intensity physical activity

Activities with an energy cost of at least 7.5 kcal/min, usually equivalent to at least slow jogging, which might be expected to leave the participant feeling out of breath and sweaty.

If the body does not use all the energy it takes in as food for physical activity, growth and maintaining

(Tables 4.4 and 4.8)

Figure 4.3

Seasonal variation in proportion of respondents with low vitamin D status (less than 25nmol/l) by sex

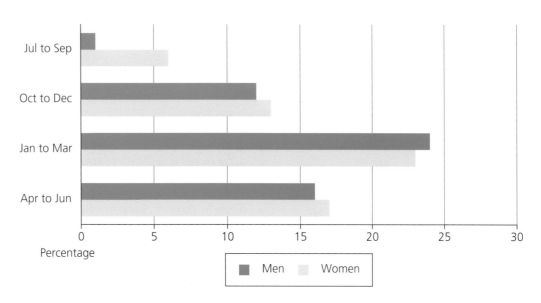

Table 4.8

Percentage distribution of plasma total cholesterol levels by sex and age of respondent

Blood analyte	Men aged (years):				All men	Women aged (years):				All women
	19–24	25–34	35–49	50–64		19–24	25–34	35–49	50–64	
	%	%	%	%	%	%	%	%	%	%
Plasma total cholesterol										
optimal level	84	59	44	41	52	83	68	52	25	52
mildly elevated level	16	31	41	37	34	17	26	41	42	35
moderately elevated level	-	7	14	20	12	-	5	6	24	10
severely elevated level	-	2	2	2	2	-	1	1	9	3

body temperature, for example, then it will be stored. Over time this will lead to an increase in body weight, which if it continues leads to an increased risk of obesity. Obesity can increase the risk of chronic diseases in later life including coronary heart disease and diabetes[24,25].

There is general consensus on the amount and type of physical activity that is beneficial to health[26,27]. The Department of Health (DH) recommendation for adults is 'At least five a week'[27]. That is:

> At least 30 minutes of physical activity on five or more days of the week. This physical activity should be of at least moderate intensity – similar to brisk walking. Activity can be taken in bouts of 10 to 15 minutes, allowing for accumulation of activity throughout the day.

The time spent in activities of moderate and vigorous/very vigorous intensity during the seven-day recording period were calculated, and added together to give the total time spent in activities of 'at least moderate intensity'. More detailed information on the physical activity methodology and calculations can be found in Volume 4[3]. Table 4.9 shows the proportion of respondents participating in at least 30 minutes of activity of at least moderate intensity by number of days and by sex and age. Figure 4.4 shows the proportion of respondents who met the physical activity recommendations by participating in at least 30 minutes of activity on five or more days of the week.

> - Overall, 36% of men and 26% of women met the DH recommendation of 'five-a-week', that is, spent 30 minutes or more in activities of at least moderate intensity on five or more days.

> - For men, the proportion who met the DH recommendation was significantly higher for those aged 19 to 24 years and 25 to 34 years than for those aged 50 to 64 years.

(Table 4.9 and Figure 4.4)

4.6 Variation by region and household receipt of benefits

This section looks at differences in physical measurements, blood pressure, blood analytes and physical activity by region and household receipt of benefits. For more detailed information on differences by these variables, *see* Volume 4[3].

4.6.1 Region[28]

Physical measurements

> - There were few significant regional differences in BMI and no clear pattern emerged for other physical measurements. However:
> - women living in the Northern region had a significantly greater waist to hip ratio than women in any other region.

Blood pressure

> - There were no regional differences in blood pressure for men or women.

Blood sample analysis

> - There were no significant regional differences in the proportions of men or women with levels of the blood analytes outside the thresholds discussed in Section 4.4.
> - There is, however, some evidence from the blood sample analyses that men and women in Scotland tended to have lower mean blood levels of some water soluble vitamins, for example, plasma vitamin C, serum folate, vitamin B_2 (EGRAC), vitamin B_6 (EAATAC) than those in other regions.

Table 4.9

Number of days per week of participation in at least 30 minutes of activity of at least moderate intensity* by sex and age of respondent

Respondents who completed physical activity diary *Percentages*

Number of days per week that 30 minutes or more per day spent in activity of at least moderate intensity	Men aged (years):				All men	Women aged (years):				All women
	19–24	25–34	35–49	50–64		19–24	25–34	35–49	50–64	
	%	%	%	%	%	%	%	%	%	%
None	21	12	20	30	21	20	14	21	24	20
One or two days a week	14	21	27	28	24	36	29	29	34	31
Three or four days a week	17	21	19	18	19	15	26	24	21	23
Five or more days a week**	49	46	34	24	36	29	30	25	22	26
Base	104	211	243	243	801	100	202	305	249	857

*   Includes moderate, vigorous and very vigorous activity.

** Participation in activities of at least moderate intensity for 30 minutes or more per day on at least five days a week is the Department of Health recommendation.

However, this was not consistent for all vitamins across all regions (data not shown, see Volume 4[3]).

Physical activity

- There were no regional differences in the proportion of men or women who met the DH recommendation for participation in physical activity.

4.6.2 Household receipt of benefits[29]

Physical measurements

- There were no significant differences in mean BMI, for men or women, living in households in receipt of benefits compared with those in non-benefit households.
- Women in benefit households had a higher mean waist to hip ratio than women in non-benefit households.

Figure 4.4

Proportion of respondents spending time on physical activity compared with the DH recommendation* by sex and age of respondent

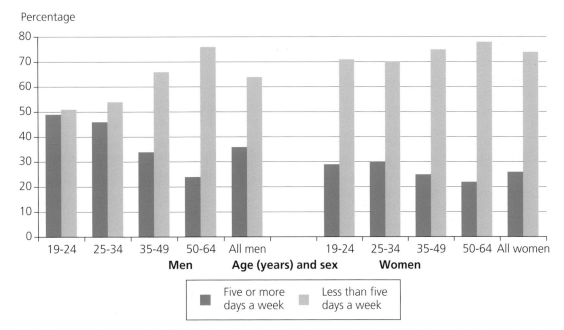

* The DH recommendation is at least 30 minutes of physical activity on five or more days of the week, of at least moderate intensity.

Blood pressure

- There were no significant differences in mean blood pressure for men or women living in households receiving benefits compared with those living in non-benefit households.

Blood sample analysis

- Respondents living in benefit households had lower mean blood levels for many nutrients compared with those in non-benefit households (*see* Volume 4[3]).
- There were few differences by household benefit status in the proportions of men and women with levels of blood analytes outside the thresholds discussed in section 4.4. For example, women living in households in receipt of benefits were more likely than those in non-benefit households to have low levels of plasma vitamin C.

Physical activity

- There were no differences by household benefit status in the proportion of men or women who met the DH recommendation for participation in physical activity.

4.7 Summary

Physical measurements

- Two-thirds of men, 66%, and over half of women, 53%, were overweight or obese, with men more likely to be overweight or obese than women (that is, BMI greater than 25).
- 25% of men and 20% of women were obese, and a further 42% of men and 32% of women were overweight.
- Men and women in the oldest age group were more likely to be classified as overweight or obese than those in the youngest age group.
- 1% of men and 3% of women, overall, were classified as underweight.
- 23% of men and 15% of women had a waist to hip ratio above the guideline thresholds.

Compared with the 1986/87 Adults Survey:

- a higher proportion of men and women were classified as overweight or obese (that is, BMI >25). 66% of men and 53% of women were overweight or obese in this survey, compared with 45% of men and 36% of women in the 1986/87 Adults survey; and

- a higher proportion of men and women were classified as obese, 25% of men and 20% of women were obese in this survey compared with 8% of men and 12% of women in the 1986/87 Adults survey.

Blood pressure

- 22% of men and 13% of women had high blood pressure, and 24% of men and 13% of women had blood pressure that is classified as 'high normal'.
- The proportions of men and women with high blood pressure increased with age.

Blood sample analysis

- 8% of women and 3% of men were anaemic, that is, they had low levels of haemoglobin in their blood.
- 11% of women and 4% of men had low levels of serum ferritin, indicating low stores of iron in the body.
- 5% of men and 3% of women had low levels of vitamin C in their blood.
- 8% of the youngest group of women and 4% of those aged 25 to 34 years had marginal folate status.
- 14% of men and 15% of women had low vitamin D status, rising to 24% of men and 28% of women in the youngest age group. Vitamin D status was lower in the winter months. For example, nearly one quarter of men and women who provided a sample in the months January to March had a 25-OHD concentration below 25nmol/l.
- 48% of men and women, overall, had blood levels of total cholesterol above the optimal level. The proportions with elevated cholesterol levels, that is above optimum, increased with age.

Physical activity

- Overall, 36% of men and 26% of women met the DH recommendation of 'five-a-week', that is, spent 30 minutes or more in activities of at least moderate intensity on five or more days.

References and endnotes

1   Gregory J, Foster K, Tyler H, Wiseman M. *The Dietary and Nutritional Survey of British Adults*. HMSO (London, 1990).

2   The Technical Report is available online at http://www.food.gov.uk/science.

   The rationale for each of the physical measurements and blood pressure, and the protocol, equipment and methodologies used are described in Appendix J of the Technical Report. The Technical Report details the procedures for obtaining and processing the blood samples (Appendix N) and describes the assay techniques and quality assurance data (Appendix O). For further details of the data editing process, data quality and the derivation of different measures of physical activity, *see* Appendix D of Volume 4 (*see* Note 3).

3   Ruston D, Hoare J, Henderson L, Gregory J, Bates CJ, Prentice A, Birch M, Swan G, Farron M. *National Diet and Nutrition Survey: adults aged 19 to 64 years. Volume 4: Nutritional status (anthropometry and blood analytes), blood pressure and physical activity*. TSO (London, 2004).

4   For more information see http://www.food.gov.uk/healthiereating/foodrelatedconditions/obesity.

5   Obesity: preventing and managing the global epidemic. Report of a WHO Consultation. Geneva, World Health Organization, 2000 (WHO Technical Report Series, No. 894).

6   Although there is no consensus on cut off points for waist to hip ratio, previous health research in England (including Health Survey for England 2001) has used ratios >=0.95 for men and >=0.85 for women based on US/Canadian guidelines (US Department of Agriculture. *Report of the dietary guidelines advisory committee on the dietary guidelines for Americans*. Washington: 1990).

7   Chalmers J *et al.* WHO-ISH Hypertension Guidelines Committee. 1999 World Health Organization – International Society of Hypertension Guidelines for the management of hypertension. *Journal of Hypertension* 1999; **17**: 151–183.

8   Thresholds for treatment intervention can be evaluated independently for systolic and diastolic blood pressure when considering elevated blood pressure levels.

9   Blood analytes not presented in this volume are: mean corpuscular volume, haematocrit, plasma iron, total iron-binding capacity, erythrocyte transketolase basal activity, plasma total homocysteine, plasma $\propto$- and β-carotene, plasma $\propto$- and β-cryptoxanthin, plasma lycopene, plasma lutein, plasma zeaxanthin, plasma $\propto$- and γ-tocopherol, plasma HDL and LDL cholesterol, plasma selenium, red cell selenium, erythrocyte glutathione peroxidase activity, plasma $\propto$1-antichymotrypsin concentration, blood mercury. For further information *see* Volume 4 (*see* Note 3).

10   World Health Organization. *Nutritional Anaemias*. Technical Report Series: 503. WHO (Geneva, 1972).

11   Bates CJ, Thurnham DI, Bingham SA, Margetts BM, Nelson M. Biochemical Markers of Nutrient Intake. In: *Design Concepts in Nutritional Epidemiology*. 2nd Edition. OUP (Oxford, 1997): 170–240.

12   Dacie JV, Lewis SM. *Practical Haematology*. 9th Edition. Churchill Livingstone (Edinburgh, 2001).

13   Sauberlich HE. Vitamin C status: methods and findings. *Ann N Y Acad Sci* 1971; **24**: 444–454.

14   Cziezel AE, Dudas I. Prevention of the first occurrence of neural tube defects by periconceptional vitamin supplementation. *N Engl J Med* 1992; **327**:1832–5.

15   Sauberlich HE, Skala JH, Dowdy RP. *Laboratory tests for the assessment of nutritional status*. CRC Press (Cleveland, Ohio, 1974).

16   Department of Health Report on Health and Social Subjects, No. **49**. *Nutrition and bone health with particular reference to calcium and vitamin D*. TSO (London, 1998).

17   Calculated as the ratio of plasma $\propto$-tocopherol to plasma total cholesterol.

18   Department of Health. Report on Health and Social Subjects: **41**. *Dietary Reference Values for Food Energy and Nutrients for the United Kingdom*. HMSO (London, 1991).

19   Department of Health. Report on Health and Social Subjects: **46**. *Nutritional Aspects of Cardiovascular Disease*. HMSO (London, 1994).

20   The British Cardiac Society, British Hyperlipidaemia Association, British Hypertension Society, endorsed by the British Diabetic Association, have issued guidance published in the article 'Joint British recommendations on prevention of coronary heart disease in clinical practice.' *Heart* 1998; **80**: 1–29.

21   Cholesterol levels were taken from non-fasting blood samples. Clinical intervention to reduce the risk of CHD is based on a full fasting lipid profile including results of total cholesterol/HDL ratio in conjunction with other risk factors by calculating the Framingham (or equivalent) score which takes all risk factors into account.

22   Health Development Agency. *Physical Activity*. Online: http://www.hda-online.org.uk/html/improving/physicalactivity.html.

23   Prior G. 'Physical Activity' In: *Health Survey for England: Cardiovascular Disease*. TSO (London, 1998).

24   National Audit Office. *Tackling obesity in England*. TSO (London, 2001).

25   National Heart Forum. *Physical activity and coronary heart disease*. Online: http://www.heartforum.org.uk/physicalactivity.html.

26   U.S. Department of Health and Human Services. *Physical activity and health: A report of the Surgeon General*. National Centre for Chronic Disease Prevention and Health Promotion (Atlanta, GA: U.S, 1994).

27   Department of Health. *At least five a week: Evidence on the impact of physical activity and its relationship to health. A report from the Chief Medical Officer*. Online: http://www.dh.gov.uk/PublicationsAndStatistics/Publications/PublicationsPolicyAndGuidance/PublicationsPolicyAndGuidanceArticle/fs/en?CONTENT_ID=4080994&chk=1Ft1Of.

28   The areas included in each of the four analysis 'regions' are given in the response chapter, Chapter 2 of the Technical Report (*see* Note 2). Definitions of 'regions' are given in the glossary (*see* Appendix F).

29   Households receiving certain benefits are those where someone in the respondent's household was currently receiving Working Families Tax Credit or had, in the previous 14 days, drawn Income Support or (Income-related) Job Seeker's Allowance. Definitions of 'household' and 'benefits (receiving)' are given in the glossary (*see* Appendix F).

Appendix A Sample design and selection

A nationally representative sample of adults aged 19 to 64 years living in private households was required. The sample was selected using a multi-stage random probability design with postal sectors as first stage units. The sampling frame included all postal sectors within mainland Great Britain; selections were made from the small users' Postcode Address File. The frame was stratified by 1991 Census variables. A total of 152 postal sectors was selected as first stage units, with probability proportional to the number of postal delivery points, and 38 sectors were allocated to each of four fieldwork waves. The allocation took account of the need to have approximately equal numbers of households in each wave of fieldwork and for each wave to be nationally representative. From each postal sector 40 addresses were randomly selected[1].

Eligibility was defined as being aged between 19 and 64 and not pregnant or breastfeeding at the time of the doorstep sift[2]. Where there was more than one adult between the ages of 19 and 64 years living in the same household, one was selected at random to take part in the survey[3]. A more detailed account of the sample design is given in Appendix D of the Technical Report[4]. In keeping with the ONS normal fieldwork procedures, a letter was sent to each household in the sample in advance of the interviewer calling, telling them briefly about the survey (*see* Appendix A of the Technical Report[4]).

As in previous surveys in the NDNS series, fieldwork covered a 12-month period, to cover any seasonality in eating behaviour and in the nutrient content of foods, for example, full fat milk. The 12-month fieldwork period was divided into four fieldwork waves, each of three months duration[5]. The fieldwork waves were:

> Wave 1: July to September 2000
> Wave 2: October to December 2000
> Wave 3: January to March 2001
> Wave 4: April to June 2001

Feasibility work carried out between September and December 1999 by the ONS and the Medical Research Council Human Nutrition Research (HNR) tested all the components of the survey and made recommendations for revisions for the mainstage. For a subgroup of the feasibility study sample, the validity of the dietary recording methodology was tested using the doubly labelled water methodology to compare energy expenditure against reported energy intake. Further details

of the design and results of the feasibility study are summarised in Appendix C of the Technical Report[4].

Because this survey, in common with other surveys in the NDNS series, includes physiological procedures which are invasive, that is a venepuncture procedure to take a blood sample, and measurements with possible clinical significance, that is venepuncture and measurement of blood pressure, it was necessary to obtain approval for the survey protocol from a Multi-centre Research Ethics Committee (MREC), and National Health Service Local Research Ethics Committees covering each of the 152 sampled areas. Further details of the ethics approval process are given in Appendix N of the Technical Report[4].

References and endnotes

[1] Initially 30 addresses were selected within each postal sector. Results from Wave 1 indicated a higher level of age-related ineligibles than expected and a much lower response rate. In order to increase the actual number of diaries completed and to give interviewers enough work an extra 10 addresses were selected for Waves 2, 3 and 4.

[2] The diet and physiology of pregnant or breastfeeding women is likely to be so different from those of other similarly aged women as to possibly distort the results. Further, as the number of pregnant or breastfeeding women identified within the overall sample of 2000 would not be adequate for analysis as a single group, it was decided that they should be regarded as ineligible for interview.

[3] Selecting only one eligible adult per household reduces the burden of the survey on the household and therefore reduces possible detrimental effects on co-operation and data quality. It also reduces the clustering of the sample associated with similar dietary behaviour within the same household and improves the precision of the estimates.

[4] The Technical Report is available online at http://www.food.gov.uk/science.

[5] As in some cases fieldwork extended beyond the end of the three-month fieldwork wave, or cases were re-allocated to another fieldwork wave, cases have been allocated to a wave for analysis purposes as follows. Any case started more than four weeks after the end of the official fieldwork wave has been allocated to the actual quarter in which it started. For example, all cases allocated to Wave 1 and started July to October 2000 appear as Wave 1 cases. Any case allocated to Wave 1 and started in November 2000 or later appears in a subsequent wave; for example a case allocated to Wave 1 which started in November 2000 is counted as Wave 2. All cases in Wave 4 (April to June 2001) had been started by the end of July 2001.

Appendix B Response and Weighting

Table B1 shows response to the dietary interview and dietary record overall and by fieldwork wave. Of the 5,673 addresses[1] issued to the interviewers, 35% were ineligible for the survey. This high rate of ineligibility is mainly due to the exclusion of those aged under 19 years and those aged 65 or over (*see* Appendix A). Just over one-third of the eligible sample, 37%, refused outright to take part in the survey. Only 2% of the eligible sample were not contacted. Overall, 61% of the eligible sample completed the dietary interview (2,251 respondents, the responding sample), including 47% who completed a full seven-day dietary record (1,724 respondents, the diary sample). Overall, 77% of those who completed the dietary interview completed a full seven-day dietary record.

Table B2 shows the proportion of respondents who consented to making a 24-hour urine collection and the proportion of cases where a sample was obtained[2]. Overall, 66% of the responding sample and 83% of the diary sample consented to making a 24-hour urine collection. A urine sample was obtained for 98% of those who consented to making the collection (65% of the responding and 81% of the diary samples).

Table B3 shows response to the physical measurements, height, weight, waist and hip circumference and blood pressure, by fieldwork wave, sex and age of respondent and the social class of the Household Reference Person. For each of these measurements, at least 77% of the responding sample and 93% of the diary sample had the measurement taken.

Table B4 shows the proportion of respondents who consented to having a blood sample taken and the proportion of cases where a sample was obtained. Overall, 63% of the responding sample and 78% of the diary sample consented to having a blood sample taken. A blood sample was obtained for 95% of those who consented (60% of the responding sample and 74% of the diary sample). In total, 1,347 blood samples were obtained.

More information on response to this survey can be found in Chapter 2 of the Technical Report[3].

While there has been a general fall in response to government social surveys over the last decade[4], the level of refusal to this NDNS was higher than expected. Steps were taken at an early stage to improve response, and included reissuing non-productive cases[5], developing the interviewer training to address further response

issues, providing general guidance on approaching and explaining the survey to respondents, and increased support to the interviewers and their managers. This met with some success so that in Wave 4 a higher proportion of the eligible sample, 67%, completed the dietary interview compared with previous waves, 56% to 60%.

Those who completed the dietary record had a similar demographic profile, by sex, age and social class of the Household Reference Person to those who completed the dietary interview (*see* also Chapter 2 of the Technical Report[3]). There were no significant differences by sex and age or by social class of the Household Reference Person in co-operation rates for the physical measurements or in the proportions consenting to a blood sample, where venepuncture was attempted and where a blood sample was obtained. However, a urine sample was obtained from a significantly lower proportion of men aged 19 to 24 years, 51% of the responding sample, and 25 to 34 years, 58%, than from those aged 35 to 49 years, 70%.

The potential for bias in any dataset increases as the level of non-response increases. Assessing bias is particularly difficult when there is little or no information on particular subgroups within the study population. An independent evaluation of the potential impact of non-response bias was undertaken by the University of Southampton[6]. The authors concluded that there was no evidence to suggest serious non-response bias, although this should be interpreted with caution as bias estimates were based upon assumptions about the total refusals and non-contacts for whom there was very little information. The authors recommended population-based weighting by sex, age and region. Indeed, without weighting for the differential response effect, estimates for different groups would be biased estimates because, in particular, they under-represent men and the youngest age group. To correct for this, the data presented in this Volume and the other volumes of this survey have been weighted using a combined weight, based on differential sampling probabilities and differential non-response. Bases in tables are weighted bases[7] scaled back to the number of cases in the responding, diary and component samples. Unweighted bases[8] are given in Tables B5 to B7. Further details of the weighting procedures are given in Appendix D of the Technical Report[3].

In summary, the estimates presented in this report result from weighting the data as effectively as possible using the available information. However,

71

results should be interpreted with caution, particularly where the sample sizes are low. The reader should note that the sample size in Scotland is particularly low and therefore standard errors may be large (*see* Appendix C for further details on standard errors).

(Tables B1 to B7)

References and endnotes

[1]   Initially 1,140 addresses were issued per wave. This was increased in Wave 2 to 1,520 addresses, 40 in each quota of work. In Wave 3, 27 addresses were withdrawn. These were unapproachable due to access restrictions in place because of the foot-and-mouth disease outbreak.

[2]   Response rates are based on those who consented to making a 24-hour urine collection, and those for whom a sample was obtained. Samples were taken from the full 24-hour collection. Not all the samples were analysed – some were damaged, or deteriorated in transit. Details of the numbers of urine samples analysed and reported on are given in Chapter 4 of Volume 3.

Henderson L, Irving K, Gregory J, Bates CJ, Prentice A, Perks J, Swan G, Farron M. *National Diet and Nutrition Survey: adults aged 19 to 64 years. Volume 3: Vitamin and mineral intake and urinary analytes.* TSO (London, 2003).

[3]   The Technical Report is available online at http://www.food.gov.uk/science.

[4]   Martin J and Matheson J. Responses to declining response rates on government surveys. *Survey Methodology Bulletin* 1999; **45**: 33–37.

[5]   Non-productive cases are those where the interviewer was unable to make contact with the selected household or respondent (non-contacts) and where the household or selected respondent refused to take part in the survey (refusals). Addresses that were returned to the office coded as refusals or non-contacts were considered for reissue. Where it was thought that a non-productive case might result in at least a dietary interview (for example, where the selected respondent had said they were too busy at the time of the original call but would be available at a later date) these addresses were issued to interviewers working in subsequent waves of fieldwork.

[6]   Skinner CJ and Holmes D (2001). *The 2000–01 National Diet and Nutrition Survey of Adults Aged 19–64 years: The Impact of Non-response.* University of Southampton. Reproduced as Appendix E of the Technical Report (*see* Note 3).

[7]   Bases presented in this report are weighted to represent the general population. These refer to the number of cases in each cell or group with the weighting factor applied (to give more or less importance to each value, according to non-response and sampling probabilities).

[8]   Unweighted bases are the original number of people in each cell or group, based on response.

Table B1

Response to the dietary interview and seven-day dietary record by wave of fieldwork*

Unweighted data

| | Wave of fieldwork | | | | | | | | All | |
| | Wave 1: July to September | | Wave 2: October to December | | Wave 3: January to March | | Wave 4: April to June | | | |
	No.	%	No.	%	No.	%	No.	%	No.	%
Set sample = 100%	1098	*100*	1397	*100*	1450	*100*	1728	*100*	5673	*100*
Ineligible	382	*35*	514	*37*	515	*36*	558	*32*	1969	*35*
Eligible sample = 100%	716	*100*	883	*100*	935	*100*	1170	*100*	3704	*100*
Non-contacts	12	*2*	24	*3*	23	*2*	30	*3*	89	*2*
Refusals	271	*38*	369	*42*	364	*39*	360	*31*	1364	*37*
Co-operation with:										
dietary interview	433	*60*	490	*56*	548	*59*	780	*67*	2251	*61*
seven-day dietary record	325	*45*	385	*44*	429	*46*	585	*50*	1724	*47*

* *For productive cases, fieldwork wave is defined as the wave (quarter) in which the dietary interview took place; for unproductive cases, fieldwork wave is the wave in which the case was issued (or reissued) (see Note 5).*

Table B2

Co-operation with the 24-hour urine collection by wave of fieldwork, sex and age of respondent and social class of household reference person

Unweighted data   Numbers and percentages

	Samples obtained*:			Consent obtained:			
	No.	As percentage of:		No.	As percentage of:		
		responding sample	diary sample		responding sample	diary sample	consenting sample
Fieldwork wave							
Wave 1	306	71	88	301	70	87	98
Wave 2	363	74	89	357	73	88	98
Wave 3	335	61	76	325	59	74	97
Wave 4	491	63	80	476	61	77	97
Sex and age of respondent							
Men aged (years)							
19–24	46	54	75	44	51	72	96
25–34	131	60	76	127	58	74	97
35–49	283	72	89	126	70	87	98
50–64	211	68	84	209	68	83	99
All	671	66	84	656	65	82	98
Women aged (years)							
19–24	67	62	74	62	57	69	92
25–34	179	65	81	175	63	80	98
35–49	332	68	83	324	66	81	98
50–64	246	66	83	242	65	82	98
All	824	66	82	803	65	80	98
Social class of household reference person							
Non-manual	843	68	83	824	66	81	98
Manual	624	66	83	605	64	81	97
All	1495	66	83	1459	65	81	98

* This includes where the respondent reported making a partial collection, that is missed at least one void during the 24 hour period, but a sample was obtained and analysed.

Table B3

Co-operation with physical measurements and blood pressure by wave of fieldwork, sex and age of respondent and social class of household reference person

Unweighted data

Numbers and percentages

Wave of fieldwork, sex and age of respondent and social class of household reference person	Height			Weight			Waist and hip circumference			Blood pressure		
	No.	As percentage of:		No.	As percentage of:		No.	As percentage of:		No.	As percentage of:	
		responding sample	diary sample		responding sample	diary sample		responding sample	diary sample		responding sample	diary sample
Fieldwork wave												
Wave 1	356	82	97	356	82	97	354	82	97	347	80	98
Wave 2	402	82	96	405	83	96	402	82	96	395	81	95
Wave 3	433	79	92	432	79	92	426	78	91	408	74	88
Wave 4	609	78	94	608	78	94	601	77	93	589	76	91
Sex and age of respondent												
Men aged (years)												
19–24	65	76	93	65	76	93	64	74	93	62	72	90
25–34	172	78	94	171	78	94	170	78	94	169	77	94
35–49	328	83	96	329	84	97	328	83	96	323	82	96
50–64	249	81	94	250	81	94	246	80	93	244	79	93
All	814	81	95	815	81	95	808	80	94	798	79	94
Women aged (years)												
19–24	83	76	87	83	76	87	82	75	87	81	74	87
25–34	216	78	95	213	77	94	213	77	94	209	75	92
35–49	393	81	96	396	81	96	387	80	94	374	77	92
50–64	294	80	94	294	80	94	293	79	94	277	75	91
All	986	79	94	986	79	94	975	78	94	941	76	91
Social class of household reference person												
Non-manual	1024	82	96	1026	82	96	1018	82	95	992	80	94
Manual	738	78	94	738	78	94	729	77	94	712	75	92
All	1800	80	95	1801	80	95	1783	79	94	1739	77	93

Table B4

Co-operation with blood sample by wave of fieldwork, sex and age of respondent and social class of household reference person

Unweighted data | Numbers and percentages

	Consent obtained:			Venepuncture attempted:				Blood sample obtained:			
	No.	As percentage of:		No.	As percentage of:			No.	As percentage of:		
		responding sample	diary sample		responding sample	diary sample	consenting sample		responding sample	diary sample	consenting sample
Fieldwork wave											
Wave 1	290	67	83	284	66	82	98	278	64	80	96
Wave 2	328	67	81	320	65	79	98	313	64	78	95
Wave 3	326	59	73	316	58	71	97	315	57	70	97
Wave 4	475	61	76	459	59	75	97	441	57	71	93
Sex and age of respondent											
Men aged (years)											
19–24	49	57	74	48	56	72	98	47	55	70	96
25–34	125	57	72	121	55	70	97	120	55	69	96
35–49	262	66	82	256	65	80	98	254	64	79	97
50–64	205	66	81	197	64	78	96	194	63	77	95
All	641	64	79	622	62	77	97	615	61	76	96
Women aged (years)											
19–24	61	56	72	58	53	70	95	53	49	64	87
25–34	163	59	74	161	58	73	99	159	57	72	98
35–49	319	66	79	313	64	77	98	306	63	75	96
50–64	235	64	79	225	61	76	96	214	58	72	91
All	778	63	77	757	61	75	98	732	59	73	94
Social class of household reference person											
Non-manual	809	65	79	785	63	77	97	771	62	76	95
Manual	579	61	77	764	60	75	132	548	58	73	95
All	1419	63	78	1379	61	76	97	1347	60	74	95

Table B5

Unweighted base numbers: dietary interview, seven-day dietary record, seven-day physical activity record and 24-hour urine collection by sex and age of respondent, region and household receipt of benefits

	Dietary interview	Seven-day weighed intake dietary record	Seven-day physical activity record	Full 24-hour urine collection*
Age				
Men aged (years)				
19–24	86	61	61	43
25–34	219	160	155	127
35–49	394	303	296	273
50–64	309	242	229	206
All	1008	766	741	649
Women aged (years)				
19–24	109	78	75	61
25–34	277	211	206	171
35–49	487	379	358	319
50–64	370	290	278	240
All	1243	958	917	791
Region				
Men				
Scotland	80	53	47	46
Northern	267	195	191	164
Central, South West and Wales	337	274	262	237
London and the South East	324	244	241	202
Women				
Scotland	111	70	69	51
Northern	341	256	248	223
Central, South West and Wales	436	350	330	281
London and the South East	355	282	270	236
Household receipt of benefits**				
Men				
Receiving benefits	145	106	102	95
Not receiving benefits	863	660	639	554
Women				
Receiving benefits	283	199	193	171
Not receiving benefits	960	759	724	620
All	2251	1724	1658	1440

* Unweighted bases are given for the number of urine samples analysed for urinary sodium excretion.

** Receipt of benefits was asked of the respondent about themselves, their partner or anyone else in the household. Benefits asked about were Working Families Tax Credit, Income Support and (Income-related) Job Seeker's Allowance.

Table B6

Unweighted base numbers: physical measurements and blood pressure by sex and age of respondent, region and household receipt of benefits

	BMI	Waist circumference	Waist to hip ratio	Blood pressure
Age				
Men aged (years)				
19–24	64	64	64	62
25–34	169	170	170	168
35–49	328	328	328	324
50–64	249	246	246	243
All	810	808	808	797
Women aged (years)				
19–24	82	82	82	80
25–34	212	213	213	210
35–49	391	387	387	373
50–64	293	293	292	276
All	978	975	974	939
Region				
Men				
Scotland	52	52	52	51
Northern	210	210	210	207
Central, South West and Wales	290	287	287	286
London and the South East	258	259	259	253
Women				
Scotland	73	71	71	70
Northern	267	264	264	254
Central, South West and Wales	349	349	348	342
London and the South East	289	291	291	273
Household receipt of benefits*				
Men				
Receiving benefits	115	115	115	116
Not receiving benefits	695	693	693	681
Women				
Receiving benefits	211	211	210	208
Not receiving benefits	767	764	764	731
All	1788	1783	1782	1736

* *Receipt of benefits was asked of the respondent about themselves, their partner or anyone else in the household. Benefits asked about were Working Families Tax Credit, Income Support and (Income-related) Job Seeker's Allowance.*

Table B7

Unweighted base numbers: blood analytes by sex and age of respondent, region and household receipt of benefits

	Blood sample*		
	Plasma retinol	Haemoglobin	Plasma iron
Age			
Men aged (years)			
19–24	45	45	45
25–34	107	119	115
35–49	213	245	243
50–64	168	191	189
All	533	600	592
Women aged (years)			
19–24	44	53	47
25–34	146	157	154
35–49	278	298	296
50–64	191	210	206
All	659	718	703
Region			
Men			
Scotland	45	45	46
Northern	140	155	148
Central, South West and Wales	191	211	214
London and the South East	157	189	184
Women			
Scotland	46	50	48
Northern	177	191	189
Central, South West and Wales	245	272	263
London and the South East	191	157	203
Household receipt of benefits**			
Men			
Receiving benefits	76	85	84
Not receiving benefits	457	515	508
Women			
Receiving benefits	149	162	159
Not receiving benefits	510	556	544
All	1192	1318	1295

* Blood analytes shown are those used to derive weighting factors for groups of analytes with similar numbers of reported results (see Appendix E).

** Receipt of benefits was asked of the respondent about themselves, their partner or anyone else in the household. Benefits asked about were Working Families Tax Credit, Income Support and (Income-related) Job Seeker's Allowance.

Appendix C Sampling errors

1   Sampling errors

This appendix examines the sources of error associated with survey estimates and refers to the calculation of standard errors and design factors. For further details on sampling errors and statistical methods refer to previous volumes in this series[1].

1.1   The accuracy of survey results

Survey results are subject to various sources of error. The total error in a survey estimate is the difference between the estimate derived from the data collected and the true value for the population. It can be thought of as being comprised of random and systematic errors, and each of these two main types of error can be subdivided into error from a number of different sources.

1.1.1   Random error

Random error is the part of the total error which would be expected to average zero if a number of repeats of the same survey were carried out based on different samples from the same population.

An important component of random error is sampling error, which arises because the estimate is based on a survey rather than a census of the population. The results of this or any other survey would be expected to vary from the true population values. The amount of variation depends on both the size of the sample and the sample design.

Random error may also arise from other sources such as the respondent's interpretation of the questions. As with all surveys carried out by the ONS, considerable efforts were made on this survey to minimise these effects through interviewer training and through feasibility work; however it is likely some will remain that are not possible to quantify.

1.1.2   Systematic error

Systematic error, or bias, applies to those sources of error that will not average to zero over a number of repeats of the survey. The category includes, for example, bias due to omission of certain parts of the population from the sampling frame, or bias due to interviewer or coder variation. A substantial effort is put into avoiding systematic errors but it is likely that some will remain.

Non-response bias is a systematic error that is of particular concern. It occurs if non-respondents to the survey, or to particular components of the survey, differ significantly in some respect from respondents, so that the responding sample is not representative of the total population. A certain level of non-response is inevitable in any voluntary survey. The resulting bias is, however, dependent not only on the absolute level of non-response, but on the extent to which non-respondents differ from respondents in terms of the measures that the survey aims to estimate.

Although respondents were encouraged to take part in all components of the survey, some refused certain components. Chapter 2 of the Technical Report[2] examines the characteristics of groups responding to the different parts of the survey package. The analysis of the sex, age and regional profile of respondents compared with population estimates showed evidence of some response bias. In particular, there was an under representation of men, and of people aged 19 to 24 years. The data for the main part of this volume (and all volumes in the series) were therefore weighted for differential non-response by sex, age and region (*see* Appendix B).

1.2   Standard errors for estimates for the NDNS of adults aged 19 to 64 years

As described in Chapter 1 and Appendix D of the Technical Report[2], this survey used a complex sample design, which involved both clustering and stratification. In considering the accuracy of estimates, standard errors calculated on the basis of a simple random sample design will be incorrect because of the complex sample design.

In a complex sample design, the size of the standard error of any estimate depends on how the characteristic of interest is spread within and between the primary sampling units (PSUs) and strata: this is taken into account by pairing adjacent PSUs from the same strata.

1.3   Estimating standard errors for other survey estimates

Although standard errors can be calculated readily by computer, there are practical problems in presenting a large number of survey estimates. One solution is to calculate standard errors for selected variables and, from these, identify design factors appropriate for the specific survey design and for different types of survey variable. The standard error of other survey measures can then be estimated using an appropriate design factor, together with the sampling error assuming a simple random sample.

1.3.1 The Design Factor (*deft*)

The effect of a complex sample design can be quantified by comparing the observed variability in the sample with the expected variability had the survey used a simple random sample. The most commonly used statistic is the design factor (*deft*) which is calculated as a ratio of the standard error for a survey estimate allowing for the full complexity of the sample design (including weighting), to the standard error assuming that the result has come from a simple random sample.

Tables B1 and B2 in Volume 1, A1 and A2 in Volume 2, and A1 to A4 in Volumes 3 and 4[1] provide standard errors and deft values, taking account of the complex sample design used on this survey, for the key variables presented in each volume for all respondents and for those who completed that component of the survey. Standard errors, and deft values, for estimates by household benefit status and region, are shown separately for men and women to reflect the way they are presented in the main part of each volume. The deft value varies between survey variables, reflecting the degree to which the characteristic is clustered within PSUs or is distributed between strata.

Overall, for age group, region and household benefit status, where geographic clustering would be expected, six out of ten of the deft values for men and eight out of ten for women are less than 1.2. Deft values of this order are considered to be small and they indicate that, in this survey, the characteristic is not markedly clustered geographically. Two of these deft values are above 1.5 for both sexes.

For the variables included in this volume, for women 69% of the deft values presented in Volumes 1 to 4 are less than 1.2, while for men 60% are less than 1.2. For women, less than 0.5% of the deft values are greater than 1.5, while for men, 4% are greater than 1.5.

1.3.2 Testing differences between means and proportions

Standard errors can be used to test whether an observed difference between two proportions or means in the sample is likely to be due to sampling error.

In testing for the significance of the differences between two survey estimates, proportions or means, the standard error calculated as for a simple random sample design was multiplied by an assumed design factor of 1.5 to allow for the complex sample design. The calculation of complex sampling errors and design factors for key characteristics show that this was a conservative estimate for some characteristics for some sex and age groups but was an optimistic estimate for other characteristics. Therefore there will be some differences in sample proportions and means which are not commented on in the text, but that are significantly different, at least at the $p<0.05$ level. Equally, there will be some differences that are described as significant in the text, but that are not significantly different when the complex sampling design is taken into account.

References and endnotes

[1] The other volumes in this series are:

(i) Henderson L, Gregory J, Swan G. *National Diet and Nutrition Survey: adults aged 19 to 64 years. Volume 1: Types and quantities of foods consumed.* TSO (London, 2002);

(ii) Henderson L, Gregory J, Irving K, Swan G. *National Diet and Nutrition Survey: adults aged 19 to 64 years. Volume 2: Energy, protein, carbohydrate, fat and alcohol intake.* TSO (London, 2003);

(iii) Henderson L, Irving K, Gregory J, Bates CJ, Prentice A, Perks J, Swan G, Farron M. *National Diet and Nutrition Survey: adults aged 19 to 64 years. Volume 3: Vitamin and mineral intake and urinary analytes.* TSO (London, 2003);

(iv) Ruston D, Hoare J, Henderson L, Gregory J, Bates CJ, Prentice A, Birch M, Swan G, Farron M. *National Diet and Nutrition Survey: adults aged 19 to 64 years. Volume 4: Nutritional status (anthropometry and blood analytes), blood pressure and physical activity.* TSO (London, 2004).

[2] The Technical Report is available online at http://www.food.gov.uk/science.

Appendix D Additional Food Consumption tables

Table D1(a)

Total quantities (grams) of food consumed in seven days by region: men**

Food category	Region								
	Scotland			Northern			Central, South West and Wales		
	Mean all	Mean consumers	% consumers	Mean all	Mean consumers	% consumers	Mean all	Mean consumers	% consumers
	g	g	%	g	g	%	g	g	%
Pasta, rice & other miscellaneous cereals***	695	774	91	500	573	87	541	637	85
Bread	871	887	98	878	881	100	897	909	99
Breakfast cereals	245	351	71	173	283	61	239	365	65
Biscuits, buns, cakes, pastries & fruit pies	213	244	88	216	267	81	310	368	84
Puddings (including dairy desserts & ice-cream)	132	283	46	116	270	43	174	325	54
Milk (whole, semi-skimmed, skimmed)	1894	2019	94	1512	1604	94	1588	1621	98
Other milk & cream	17	*	26	50	224	22	47	143	33
Cheese	115	147	78	109	145	75	115	150	77
Yogurt & fromage frais	147	*	32	173	492	35	100	328	31
Eggs & egg dishes	166	229	72	131	188	70	180	247	73
Fats & oils	102	110	94	109	114	95	120	125	96
Meat, meat dishes & meat products	1544	1544	100	1441	1456	99	1360	1386	98
Fish & fish dishes	254	346	74	205	297	69	212	311	68
Vegetables & vegetable dishes (excluding potatoes)	861	861	100	916	923	100	929	939	99
Potatoes	895	937	95	811	815	100	877	891	98
Savoury snacks	36	*	40	56	103	54	62	100	62
Fruit (excluding fruit juice)	765	899	86	555	764	73	557	771	72
Nuts	15	*	9	11	67	16	19	92	21
Sugars, preserves & sweet spreads	119	182	66	142	201	71	152	187	81
Confectionery	62	121	52	86	138	62	91	148	61
Fruit juice	327	706	46	287	823	35	286	712	40
Soft drinks, not low calorie	904	1515	60	960	1698	56	1252	1825	68
Soft drinks, low calorie	824	*	43	597	1823	33	578	1637	35
Alcoholic drinks	3079	3850	80	4186	5013	83	3265	4059	80
Tea, coffee & water†	6276	6276	100	6750	6861	98	7070	7070	100
Miscellaneous††	521	548	95	344	356	97	370	379	98
Base = number of respondents			65			234			294

*   Number of consumers is less than 30 and too small to calculate mean values reliably.
**   Data shown in this table may differ from data presented in Table 2.12(a) of Volume 1 due to an error in the application of the dilution factor.
       Revised Volume 1 tables are available online at www.food.gov.uk.
***   Pasta, rice & other miscellaneous cereals includes pizza.
†   Water includes tap water & bottled water, without added sugar or artificial sweeteners. Tea and coffee amounts are as consumed.
††   Includes powdered beverages (except tea & coffee), soups, sauces, condiments & artificial sweeteners.

London and the South East			All men			Food category
Mean all	Mean consumers	% consumers	Mean all	Mean consumers	% consumers	
g	g	%	g	g	%	
698	738	95	587	661	89	Pasta, rice & other miscellaneous cereals***
781	790	99	856	865	99	Bread
242	382	63	222	347	64	Breakfast cereals
258	316	82	261	315	83	Biscuits, buns, cakes, pastries & fruit pies
153	318	48	149	306	49	Puddings (including dairy desserts & ice-cream)
1345	1485	91	1521	1609	94	Milk (whole, semi-skimmed, skimmed)
65	187	35	51	169	30	Other milk & cream
132	156	84	118	150	79	Cheese
132	380	35	134	403	33	Yogurt & fromage frais
152	226	67	157	223	70	Eggs & egg dishes
87	93	93	106	112	95	Fats & oils
1364	1428	95	1398	1430	98	Meat, meat dishes & meat products
229	325	71	218	314	70	Fish & fish dishes
1071	1087	99	961	971	99	Vegetables & vegetable dishes (excluding potatoes)
742	766	97	821	837	98	Potatoes
63	119	53	58	106	55	Savoury snacks
677	855	79	607	806	75	Fruit (excluding fruit juice)
21	73	29	17	81	21	Nuts
109	142	77	134	177	76	Sugars, preserves & sweet spreads
92	152	61	87	144	61	Confectionery
456	876	52	339	795	43	Fruit juice
1017	1522	67	1075	1680	64	Soft drinks, not low calorie
558	1664	34	597	1721	35	Soft drinks, low calorie
3227	4145	78	3498	4345	81	Alcoholic drinks
6806	6966	98	6842	6919	99	Tea, coffee & water[†]
444	475	93	396	413	96	Miscellaneous[††]
		240			833	Base = number of respondents

Table D1(b)

Total quantities (grams) of food consumed in seven days by region: women**

Food category	Region								
	Scotland			Northern			Central, South West and Wales		
	Mean all	Mean consumers	% consumers	Mean all	Mean consumers	% consumers	Mean all	Mean consumers	% consumers
	g	g	%	g	g	%	g	g	%
Pasta, rice & other miscellaneous cereals***	490	559	88	389	456	86	377	459	82
Bread	511	543	94	580	586	99	575	586	98
Breakfast cereals	203	266	76	178	252	71	181	262	69
Biscuits, buns, cakes, pastries & fruit pies	169	198	85	187	230	81	213	252	85
Puddings (including dairy desserts & ice-cream)	162	301	53	125	242	52	139	254	55
Milk (whole, semi-skimmed, skimmed)	1281	1414	91	1414	1486	95	1382	1472	94
Other milk & cream	48	*	21	54	192	28	43	136	32
Cheese	107	140	76	91	125	73	97	129	76
Yogurt & fromage frais	168	*	41	198	459	43	163	377	43
Eggs & egg dishes	105	168	62	111	163	69	104	160	65
Fats & oils	58	64	89	66	72	91	69	75	93
Meat, meat dishes & meat products	911	966	94	851	920	93	904	964	94
Fish & fish dishes	200	253	79	213	289	74	188	256	73
Vegetables & vegetable dishes (excluding potatoes)	727	735	98	848	852	100	903	920	98
Potatoes	611	663	92	659	664	100	703	725	97
Savoury snacks	44	76	58	44	79	55	44	76	58
Fruit (excluding fruit juice)	847	946	89	685	885	78	680	801	85
Nuts	5	*	12	6	46	14	10	53	20
Sugars, preserves & sweet spreads	61	88	70	83	123	68	92	134	68
Confectionery	90	115	79	72	131	55	80	118	68
Fruit juice	491	910	53	265	598	45	318	703	45
Soft drinks, not low calorie	711	1135	62	664	1147	58	800	1440	56
Soft drinks, low calorie	1138	2383	47	663	1511	44	633	1480	43
Alcoholic drinks	825	1186	70	1285	1957	66	879	1311	67
Tea, coffee & water†	6208	6315	98	7042	7106	99	7000	7020	100
Miscellaneous††	551	593	92	390	402	97	317	329	97
Base = number of respondents			66			229			327

* Number of consumers is less than 30 and too small to calculate mean values reliably.
** Data shown in this table may differ from data presented in Table 2.12(b) of Volume 1 due to an error in the application of the dilution factor. Revised Volume 1 tables are available online at www.food.gov.uk.
*** Pasta, rice & other miscellaneous cereals includes pizza.
† Water includes tap water & bottled water, without added sugar or artificial sweeteners. Tea and coffee amounts are as consumed.
†† Includes powdered beverages (except tea & coffee), soups, sauces, condiments & artificial sweeteners.

London and the South East			All women			Food category
Mean all	Mean consumers	% consumers	Mean all	Mean consumers	% consumers	
g	g	%	g	g	%	
524	605	87	433	511	85	Pasta, rice & other miscellaneous cereals***
556	565	99	566	576	98	Bread
195	285	69	186	267	70	Breakfast cereals
216	250	87	204	242	84	Biscuits, buns, cakes, pastries & fruit pies
134	243	55	135	251	54	Puddings (including dairy desserts & ice-cream)
1256	1365	92	1345	1440	93	Milk (whole, semi-skimmed, skimmed)
79	216	37	57	181	32	Other milk & cream
94	122	77	96	127	75	Cheese
158	373	43	171	399	43	Yogurt & fromage frais
121	190	64	111	170	65	Eggs & egg dishes
68	76	90	67	74	91	Fats & oils
836	931	90	870	943	92	Meat, meat dishes & meat products
255	359	71	216	294	73	Fish & fish dishes
1069	1074	100	926	935	99	Vegetables & vegetable dishes (excluding potatoes)
594	622	96	652	674	97	Potatoes
47	86	56	45	80	57	Savoury snacks
768	927	83	720	871	83	Fruit (excluding fruit juice)
22	78	28	12	62	20	Nuts
64	92	69	79	115	68	Sugars, preserves & sweet spreads
71	111	64	76	118	64	Confectionery
353	708	50	327	697	47	Fruit juice
613	1152	53	702	1254	56	Soft drinks, not low calorie
723	1784	41	705	1650	43	Soft drinks, low calorie
858	1247	69	973	1444	67	Alcoholic drinks
6954	7037	99	6938	6996	99	Tea, coffee & water[†]
311	335	93	351	369	95	Miscellaneous[††]
		268			891	Base = number of respondents

87

Table D2(a)

Total quantities (grams) of food consumed in seven days by whether someone in the respondent's household was receiving certain benefits: men**

Food category	Whether receiving benefits						All men		
	Receiving benefits			Not receiving benefits					
	Mean all	Mean consumers	% consumers	Mean all	Mean consumers	% consumers	Mean all	Mean consumers	% consumers
	g	g	%	g	g	%	g	g	%
Pasta, rice & other miscellaneous cereals***	534	604	88	595	670	89	587	661	89
Bread	836	861	97	859	865	99	856	865	99
Breakfast cereals	150	290	52	233	353	66	222	347	64
Biscuits, buns, cakes, pastries & fruit pies	196	253	77	270	324	84	261	315	83
Puddings (including dairy desserts & ice-cream)	111	324	35	154	304	51	149	306	49
Milk (whole, semi-skimmed, skimmed)	1405	1487	95	1538	1628	94	1521	1609	94
Other milk & cream	29	*	23	54	174	31	51	169	30
Cheese	96	139	69	121	152	80	118	150	79
Yogurt & fromage frais	57	*	21	145	414	35	134	403	33
Eggs & egg dishes	163	231	71	156	222	70	157	223	70
Fats & oils	105	110	95	106	112	95	106	112	95
Meat, meat dishes & meat products	1405	1437	97	1398	1429	98	1398	1430	98
Fish & fish dishes	195	296	66	222	317	70	218	314	70
Vegetables & vegetable dishes (excluding potatoes)	844	853	99	979	989	99	961	971	99
Potatoes	870	892	97	813	829	98	821	837	98
Savoury snacks	54	122	45	59	104	57	58	106	55
Fruit (excluding fruit juice)	402	678	59	639	821	78	607	806	75
Nuts	16	*	10	17	77	23	17	81	21
Sugars, preserves & sweet spreads	173	215	80	129	171	75	134	177	76
Confectionery	97	168	57	86	141	61	87	144	61
Fruit juice	189	681	28	361	806	45	339	795	43
Soft drinks, not low calorie	1300	1928	67	1040	1640	63	1075	1680	64
Soft drinks, low calorie	414	1137	36	625	1814	34	597	1721	35
Alcoholic drinks	2090	3607	58	3712	4422	84	3498	4345	81
Tea, coffee & water†	6447	6685	96	6902	6954	99	6842	6919	99
Miscellaneous††	324	356	91	407	421	97	396	413	96
Base = number of respondents			110			723			833

* Number of consumers is less than 30 and too small to calculate mean values reliably.
** Data shown in this table may differ from data presented in Table 2.13(a) of Volume 1 due to an error in the application of the dilution factor. Revised Volume 1 tables are available online at www.food.gov.uk.
*** Pasta, rice & other miscellaneous cereals includes pizza.
† Water includes tap water & bottled water, without added sugar or artificial sweeteners. Tea and coffee amounts are as consumed.
†† Includes powdered beverages (except tea & coffee), soups, sauces, condiments & artificial sweeteners.

Table D2(b)

Total quantities (grams) of food consumed in seven days by whether someone in the respondent's household was receiving certain benefits: women**

| Food category | Whether receiving benefits | | | | | | All women | | |
| | Receiving benefits | | | Not receiving benefits | | | | | |
	Mean all	Mean consumers	% consumers	Mean all	Mean consumers	% consumers	Mean all	Mean consumers	% consumers
	g	g	%	g	g	%	g	g	%
Pasta, rice & other miscellaneous cereals***	534	524	77	595	508	86	433	511	85
Bread	836	544	95	859	583	99	566	576	98
Breakfast cereals	150	217	58	233	275	72	186	267	70
Biscuits, buns, cakes, pastries & fruit pies	196	213	73	270	247	87	204	242	84
Puddings (including dairy desserts & ice-cream)	111	206	38	154	257	57	135	251	54
Milk (whole, semi-skimmed, skimmed)	1405	1443	90	1538	1439	94	1345	1440	93
Other milk & cream	29	*	18	54	174	34	57	181	32
Cheese	96	115	63	121	129	78	96	127	75
Yogurt & fromage frais	57	283	28	145	413	46	171	399	43
Eggs & egg dishes	163	160	62	156	172	66	111	170	65
Fats & oils	105	68	87	106	75	92	67	74	91
Meat, meat dishes & meat products	1405	970	96	1398	938	91	870	943	92
Fish & fish dishes	195	252	62	222	302	75	216	294	73
Vegetables & vegetable dishes (excluding potatoes)	844	691	97	979	983	99	926	935	99
Potatoes	870	668	94	813	675	97	652	674	97
Savoury snacks	54	85	61	59	78	56	45	80	57
Fruit (excluding fruit juice)	402	633	67	639	908	86	720	871	83
Nuts	16	*	14	17	57	21	12	62	20
Sugars, preserves & sweet spreads	173	171	69	129	104	68	79	115	68
Confectionery	97	117	55	86	119	66	76	118	64
Fruit juice	189	851	39	361	672	49	327	697	47
Soft drinks, not low calorie	1300	1459	59	1040	1210	55	702	1254	56
Soft drinks, low calorie	414	1180	35	625	1724	44	705	1650	43
Alcoholic drinks	2090	2056	55	3712	1347	70	973	1444	67
Tea, coffee & water†	6447	6424	99	6902	7111	99	6938	6996	99
Miscellaneous††	324	292	91	407	384	96	351	369	95
Base = number of respondents			150			741			891

*　　　Number of consumers is less than 30 and too small to calculate mean values reliably.

**　　Data shown in this table may differ from data presented in Table 2.13(b) of Volume 1 due to an error in the application of the dilution factor. Revised Volume 1 tables are available online at www.food.gov.uk.

***　Pasta, rice & other miscellaneous cereals includes pizza.

†　　　Water includes tap water & bottled water, without added sugar or artificial sweeteners. Tea and coffee amounts are as consumed.

††　　Includes powdered beverages (except tea & coffee), soups, sauces, condiments & artificial sweeteners.

Table D3(a)

Comparison of total quantities (grams) of food consumed in seven days in two surveys: 1986/87 Adults Survey; 2000/01 NDNS Adults aged 19 to 64 years: men

Type of food	Men aged (years):												All men		
	1986/87 Adults Survey**														
	16–24			25–34			35–49			50–64					
	Mean all	Mean consum-ers	% consum-ers	Mean all	Mean consum-ers	% consum-ers	Mean all	Mean consum-ers	% consum-ers	Mean all	Mean consum-ers	% consum-ers	Mean all	Mean consum-ers	% consum-ers
	g	g	%	g	g	%	g	g	%	g	g	%	g	g	%
Pasta, rice & other															
miscellaneous cereals	325	438	74	347	426	82	275	383	72	178	294	60	277	387	72
of which:															
Pasta	60	257	23	102	313	33	70	268	26	36	234	15	67	275	25
Rice	150	416	36	152	324	47	125	358	35	79	325	24	124	353	35
Bread	924	932	99	878	889	99	965	965	100	959	959	100	935	940	100
of which:															
White bread	677	751	90	531	595	89	606	683	89	554	649	85	590	668	88
Wholemeal bread	183	490	37	244	481	51	269	522	51	284	546	52	250	514	49
Breakfast cereals	125	246	51	138	233	59	190	346	55	183	300	61	163	288	57
Biscuits, buns, cakes,															
pastries & fruit pies	281	344	82	290	326	89	400	444	90	408	444	92	353	398	89
of which:															
Biscuits	90	149	60	104	134	78	104	141	74	113	141	80	104	141	74
Fruit pies	34	168	20	34	170	20	44	174	25	55	199	28	42	179	24
Buns, cakes & pastries	157	255	62	151	224	68	253	325	78	239	307	78	207	286	72
Puddings (including dairy															
desserts & ice cream)	218	398	55	229	364	63	267	385	69	303	422	72	257	392	66
of which:															
Ice cream	31	149	21	171	58	34	49	137	36	58	144	40	50	148	34
Milk****	1663	1736	96	1730	1772	98	1681	1768	95	1777	1830	97	1713	1779	96
of which:															
Whole milk	1324	1515	87	1320	1421	93	1177	1335	88	1337	1533	87	1280	1440	89
Semi-skimmed milk	264	1485	18	269	1290	21	300	1367	22	258	1195	22	275	1324	21
Skimmed milk	75	*	10	141	966	15	204	1196	17	181	1032	18	158	1036	15
Cheese	106	145	73	124	161	77	147	174	85	146	171	85	134	165	81
of which:															
Cottage cheese	1	*	1	4	*	5	4	*	4	7	108	7	4	104	4
Other cheese	106	144	73	121	159	76	143	169	85	139	165	84	129	161	80
Yogurt & fromage frais	64	296	22	69	304	23	64	303	21	42	243	17	60	289	21
Eggs & egg dishes	178	239	74	191	238	80	193	223	87	182	215	85	187	227	82
Fats & oils	132	141	94	136	139	98	160	161	99	171	176	97	151	156	97
of which:															
Butter	38	81	46	43	69	61	50	85	59	69	116	60	51	88	57
Meat & meat products	1389	1408	99	1367	1384	99	1232	1246	99	1177	1177	100	1280	1292	99
of which:															
Bacon & ham	131	172	76	119	155	77	135	165	82	159	184	86	137	169	81
Beef, veal & dishes	261	351	74	361	468	77	325	393	83	274	333	82	308	387	80
Lamb & dishes	69	210	33	69	237	29	60	183	33	96	248	39	73	218	33
Pork & dishes	67	161	42	96	211	46	75	182	41	93	189	49	83	187	44
Coated chicken & turkey	15	*	9	20	152	13	15	*	8	6	156	4	14	169	8
Chicken & turkey dishes	193	292	66	205	294	70	183	271	68	157	246	64	184	275	67
Liver, liver products & dishes	17	119	14	29	129	22	35	124	28	34	133	25	30	127	23
Burgers & kebabs	127	262	49	84	206	41	37	142	26	20	133	15	61	197	31
Sausages	119	196	61	96	172	56	94	156	60	85	158	54	97	168	58
Meat pies & pastries	267	371	72	173	293	59	158	275	58	134	251	53	177	297	60
Other meat & meat products	123	276	44	116	237	49	114	228	50	122	215	56	118	235	50

NDNS adults aged 19 to 64, Volume 5 2004

2000/01 NDNS***												All men			Type of food
19–24			25–34			35–49			50–64						
Mean all	Mean consumers	% consumers	Mean all	Mean consumers	% consumers	Mean all	Mean consumers	% consumers	Mean all	Mean consumers	% consumers	Mean all	Mean consumers	% consumers	
g	g	%	g	g	%	g	g	%	g	g	%	g	g	%	
767	802	96	743	807	92	564	635	89	397	480	83	587	661	89	Pasta, rice & other miscellaneous cereals
															of which:
280	425	66	266	463	58	198	382	52	151	356	42	212	406	52	Pasta
211	394	54	280	476	59	243	418	58	171	373	46	226	420	54	Rice
727	743	98	862	870	99	883	892	99	879	885	99	856	865	99	Bread
															of which:
565	600	94	570	610	94	604	639	94	566	629	90	578	623	93	White bread
54	*	19	131	450	29	136	376	36	146	363	40	127	381	33	Wholemeal bread
108	220	49	230	355	65	205	309	66	280	416	67	222	347	64	Breakfast cereals
167	218	77	216	268	81	268	327	82	332	379	88	261	315	83	Biscuits, buns, cakes, pastries & fruit pies
															of which:
65	132	49	90	145	62	101	157	64	104	150	70	95	149	63	Biscuits
6	*	5	20	138	14	20	*	12	37	184	20	23	165	14	Fruit pies
97	193	50	106	200	53	147	246	60	191	295	65	143	246	58	Buns, cakes & pastries
92	301	31	119	291	41	156	277	56	191	346	55	149	306	49	Puddings (including dairy desserts & ice cream)
															of which:
27	*	17	42	179	23	49	151	32	52	176	29	45	166	27	Ice cream
933	1030	91	1541	1605	96	1670	1730	96	1605	1731	92	1521	1609	94	Milk****
															of which:
130	*	19	421	997	42	426	1190	36	384	996	38	373	1031	36	Whole milk
755	983	77	902	1163	78	1095	1435	76	1015	1503	68	976	1318	74	Semi-skimmed milk
48	*	5	218	*	12	150	910	17	206	1082	19	172	1171	15	Skimmed milk
94	150	63	119	151	79	119	148	80	126	152	83	118	150	79	Cheese
															of which:
0	-	-	3	*	2	5	*	3	7	*	4	4	*	3	Cottage cheese
94	150	63	116	147	79	114	144	79	120	145	82	114	146	78	Other cheese
90	309	29	123	419	29	141	423	33	154	404	38	134	403	33	Yogurt & fromage frais
129	266	49	153	218	70	145	200	72	185	237	78	157	223	70	Eggs & egg dishes
105	112	94	96	102	94	102	109	94	119	123	96	106	112	95	Fats & oils
															of which:
24	66	37	14	38	38	28	66	42	34	83	40	26	64	40	Butter
1438	1459	99	1462	1482	99	1439	1481	97	1286	1322	97	1398	1430	98	Meat & meat products
															of which:
125	187	67	128	165	78	133	171	78	153	188	81	137	177	77	Bacon & ham
315	483	66	302	431	70	299	441	68	281	423	66	296	438	68	Beef, veal & dishes
45	*	24	73	333	22	58	262	22	62	217	29	61	253	24	Lamb & dishes
39	*	19	69	216	32	87	235	37	95	246	39	79	231	34	Pork & dishes
85	222	39	62	201	31	58	216	26	24	181	13	52	207	25	Coated chicken & turkey
345	436	80	405	501	81	419	526	79	334	386	86	380	463	82	Chicken & turkey dishes
3	*	5	12	*	10	19	143	13	21	139	15	15	133	12	Liver, liver products & dishes
192	295	66	128	292	44	73	232	32	15	*	11	86	261	33	Burgers & kebabs
121	222	55	96	166	58	98	167	58	75	154	49	93	170	55	Sausages
131	328	40	139	298	47	137	291	47	148	306	48	140	302	46	Meat pies & pastries
37	135	28	49	187	26	58	184	32	78	212	36	59	189	31	Other meat & meat products

Type of food	Men aged (years):														
	1986/87 Adults Survey**												All men		
	16–24			25–34			35–49			50–64					
	Mean all	Mean consum-ers	% consum-ers	Mean all	Mean consum-ers	% consum-ers	Mean all	Mean consum-ers	% consum-ers	Mean all	Mean consum-ers	% consum-ers	Mean all	Mean consum-ers	% consum-ers
	g	g	%	g	g	%	g	g	%	g	g	%	g	g	%
Fish & fish dishes	164	246	67	194	270	72	229	293	78	247	298	83	213	281	76
of which:															
White fish	121	220	55	136	231	59	143	222	65	160	231	69	142	226	63
Oily fish†	31	135	23	49	145	34	60	172	35	76	181	42	56	164	34
Shellfish	12	*	10	9	*	10	26	175	15	10	92	11	15	129	12
Vegetables & vegetable dishes															
(excluding potatoes)	832	836	100	1000	1020	98	1139	1139	100	1137	1137	100	1046	1051	99
of which:															
Raw carrots	8	*	8	8	69	12	9	68	14	9	69	14	9	73	12
Other raw & salad vegetables	71	119	59	115	157	73	130	179	73	133	189	71	116	166	70
Raw tomatoes	61	124	49	96	144	67	117	167	70	139	191	73	107	162	66
Peas	130	178	73	130	170	76	140	200	70	118	163	72	130	179	73
Green beans	17	105	16	24	104	23	35	144	25	28	122	23	27	123	22
Baked beans	182	302	60	142	271	52	125	233	54	75	186	40	128	249	51
Leafy green vegetables	83	173	48	99	178	56	126	191	66	164	229	72	121	197	61
Carrots - not raw	64	117	55	70	130	54	87	133	66	93	137	68	80	131	61
Tomatoes - not raw	9	*	10	16	85	19	18	80	22	42	138	30	21	102	21
Other vegetables	208	263	79	301	347	87	352	378	93	336	365	92	308	347	89
Potatoes	1201	1213	99	1052	1082	97	1086	1099	99	1014	1029	99	1083	1100	98
of which:															
Potato chips	567	629	90	418	501	84	329	405	81	220	315	70	369	458	81
Fried/roast potatoes & fried															
potato products	133	257	52	125	233	54	141	242	58	117	216	54	129	237	55
Potato products, not fried	4	*	3	6	*	5	3	*	2	4	109	4	4	116	4
Other potatoes & potato dishes	498	566	88	504	590	85	614	661	93	673	720	93	580	643	90
Savoury snacks	80	117	69	60	102	59	34	77	44	20	64	31	45	93	49
Fruit (excluding fruit juice)	253	400	63	430	607	71	504	653	77	596	720	83	460	619	74
of which:															
Apples & pears	98	256	38	177	383	46	226	403	56	241	416	58	193	381	51
Citrus fruit	43	241	18	71	270	26	62	273	23	59	207	29	60	248	24
Bananas	38	204	19	53	207	26	59	227	26	68	200	34	56	211	27
Canned fruit in juice	3	*	4	12	*	9	13	*	8	19	158	12	12	147	8
Canned fruit in syrup	19	138	14	23	150	15	36	170	21	41	193	21	31	168	19
Other fruit	52	240	22	94	266	35	107	285	38	168	332	51	108	292	37
Nuts	3	*	8	8	59	13	8	61	13	9	73	13	7	60	12
Sugars, preserves & sweet spreads	159	196	81	188	214	88	228	259	88	240	283	85	208	242	86
of which:															
Table sugar	135	180	75	159	211	75	180	252	72	176	249	71	165	227	73
Preserves	23	84	28	27	66	41	47	86	54	61	105	58	41	88	47
Sweet spreads, fillings & icings	1	*	3	2	*	6	1	*	5	3	32	8	2	28	6
Confectionery	118	178	66	88	141	62	55	104	53	45	100	45	73	130	56
of which:															
Sugar confectionery	15	70	22	7	46	16	9	53	17	9	60	15	10	57	17
Chocolate confectionery	103	179	58	81	139	58	46	99	47	36	94	39	63	127	50
Fruit juice	313	745	42	322	718	45	233	619	38	181	556	33	257	659	39
Soft drinks, not low calorie††	1592	1981	80	788	1151	69	525	967	54	359	759	47	755	1238	61
Soft drinks, low calorie††	85	*	11	159	1124	14	80	671	12	109	*	8	107	934	11

2000/01 NDNS***												All men			Type of food
19–24			25–34			35–49			50–64						
Mean all	Mean consumers	% consumers	Mean all	Mean consumers	% consumers	Mean all	Mean consumers	% consumers	Mean all	Mean consumers	% consumers	Mean all	Mean consumers	% consumers	
g	g	%	g	g	%	g	g	%	g	g	%	g	g	%	
130	280	46	159	260	61	229	312	74	297	359	83	218	314	70	Fish & fish dishes
															of which:
86	221	39	80	219	37	105	217	48	164	272	60	114	239	48	White fish
23	*	18	64	195	33	97	215	45	105	194	54	81	198	41	Oily fish†
20	*	8	15	105	15	28	122	23	28	148	19	24	135	18	Shellfish
															Vegetables & vegetable dishes
665	691	96	854	866	99	1006	1008	100	1135	1140	100	961	971	99	(excluding potatoes)
															of which:
5	*	5	9	*	9	9	69	13	13	70	18	10	78	12	Raw carrots
78	107	73	121	153	79	137	184	75	150	197	76	129	170	76	Other raw & salad vegetables
55	97	56	96	157	61	106	159	66	138	180	77	106	159	67	Raw tomatoes
49	117	42	70	130	53	94	152	62	115	172	67	88	150	59	Peas
11	*	15	11	*	13	22	106	21	42	136	31	24	113	21	Green beans
241	503	48	135	256	53	150	312	48	104	233	44	144	299	48	Baked beans
30	102	30	46	125	36	76	139	55	121	188	64	76	153	49	Leafy green vegetables
40	81	50	51	104	49	63	112	57	79	119	67	62	109	57	Carrots - not raw
6	*	7	32	154	21	36	126	28	54	157	34	37	143	26	Tomatoes - not raw
149	210	71	283	342	83	312	357	87	319	371	86	286	341	84	Other vegetables
864	864	100	777	796	98	811	830	98	850	868	98	821	837	98	Potatoes
															of which:
455	528	86	319	415	77	289	380	76	233	341	68	302	401	75	Potato chips
															Fried/roast potatoes & fried potato products
92	269	34	95	240	40	94	217	43	111	244	46	99	237	42	
22	*	8	12	*	9	10	*	6	11	*	8	13	167	8	Potato products, not fried
295	411	72	351	442	79	418	495	85	494	547	90	407	489	83	Other potatoes & potato dishes
92	146	63	75	112	66	58	101	57	31	76	40	58	106	55	Savoury snacks
190	410	46	428	633	68	694	834	83	855	987	87	607	806	75	Fruit (excluding fruit juice)
															of which:
76	251	31	158	393	40	242	444	55	296	498	59	215	437	49	Apples & pears
14	*	10	53	265	20	103	350	29	91	292	31	75	299	25	Citrus fruit
71	*	25	129	312	42	210	381	55	229	390	59	176	363	49	Bananas
2	*	1	7	*	5	16	134	12	30	253	12	16	183	9	Canned fruit in juice
8	*	4	2	*	0	13	*	7	24	*	9	13	236	6	Canned fruit in syrup
19	*	8	79	285	28	110	258	43	185	354	52	113	303	37	Other fruit
1	*	8	22	93	24	20	81	24	17	82	21	17	81	21	Nuts
91	112	82	122	162	75	146	200	73	152	198	77	134	177	76	Sugars, preserves & sweet spreads
															of which:
77	108	72	105	167	63	118	204	58	105	193	55	106	176	60	Table sugar
12	*	18	12	45	26	26	69	38	46	93	49	26	74	36	Preserves
2	*	12	5	*	8	1	*	6	1	*	4	2	34	7	Sweet spreads, fillings & icings
133	202	66	95	141	67	95	145	66	54	114	47	87	144	61	Confectionery
															of which:
26	*	20	10	49	21	19	77	24	10	64	15	15	73	20	Sugar confectionery
107	171	62	84	138	61	76	131	58	45	108	42	73	134	54	Chocolate confectionery
264	792	33	258	632	41	393	929	42	385	798	48	339	795	43	Fruit juice
2662	2848	94	1336	1701	79	766	1314	58	478	1076	44	1075	1680	64	Soft drinks, not low calorie††
565	1660	34	837	2113	40	612	1547	40	388	1500	26	597	1721	35	Soft drinks, low calorie††

Type of food	Men aged (years): 1986/87 Adults Survey**												All men		
	16–24			25–34			35–49			50–64					
	Mean all	Mean consumers	% consumers	Mean all	Mean consumers	% consumers	Mean all	Mean consumers	% consumers	Mean all	Mean consumers	% consumers	Mean all	Mean consumers	% consumers
	g	g	%	g	g	%	g	g	%	g	g	%	g	g	%
Alcoholic drinks	3734	5832	64	3997	4928	81	3931	4893	80	2923	3817	77	3654	4786	76
of which:															
Liqueurs	1	*	2	1	*	2	2	*	3	2	*	3	2	60	3
Spirits	11	*	12	22	128	17	57	205	28	66	190	34	42	176	24
Wine†††	53	363	15	153	484	32	229	639	36	208	590	35	171	562	31
Fortified wine	9	*	2	14	*	7	32	299	11	42	246	17	26	266	10
Beer & lager†††	3488	6068	58	3652	5125	71	3512	5128	69	2561	4481	57	3301	5148	64
Cider & perry†††	172	*	10	156	1162	13	100	1077	9	44	*	7	113	1158	10
Tea & water††††	4054	4171	97	5975	6071	98	6828	6848	100	6769	6769	100	6068	6130	99
Base			214			254			346			273			1087

*   Numbers of consumers too small to calculate mean/standard deviation values reliably.

**   Gregory JR et al. The Dietary and Nutritional Survey of British Adults. HMSO (London, 1990)
Food consumption data from the 1986/87 Adults Survey has been recalculated, and the data for both surveys restructured into specific food groups to allow comparisons to be made. Consequently, there may be small discrepancies between the 1986/87 data as published in 1990 and that presented in this volume.

*** Data shown in this table may differ from data presented in Tables 2.10(a) and 2.11(a) of Volume 1 due to an error in the application of the dilution factor. Revised Volume 1 tables are available online at www.food.gov.uk.

**** Includes whole milk, semi-skimmed milk and skimmed milk only. Other milks and creams excluded as data are not comparable between the two surveys due to differences in the dietary recording methodology.

†   Oily fish includes canned tuna.

††   Figures for soft drinks, low calorie and not low calorie, are as consumed, that is includes concentrated drinks plus diluent.

††† Includes low-alcohol variations.

†††† Water includes tap water, and bottled water without added sugar or artificial sweeteners; coffee is excluded from this table as data between the two surveys on consumption of coffee are not comparable due to differences in dietary recording methodology.

NDNS adults aged 19 to 64, Volume 5 2004

2000/01 NDNS***												All men			Type of food
19–24			25–34			35–49			50–64						
Mean all	Mean consum-ers	% consum-ers	Mean all	Mean consum-ers	% consum-ers	Mean all	Mean consum-ers	% consum-ers	Mean all	Mean consum-ers	% consum-ers	Mean all	Mean consum-ers	% consum-ers	
g	g	%	g	g	%	g	g	%	g	g	%	g	g	%	
3622	4543	80	3994	4878	82	3530	4201	84	2983	3917	76	3498	4345	81	Alcoholic drinks
															of which:
1	*	2	4	*	3	3	*	3	4	*	3	3	*	3	Liqueurs
16	*	21	19	*	11	50	242	21	52	214	25	38	197	19	Spirits
101	*	19	236	784	30	390	898	43	455	1091	42	332	914	36	Wine†††
10	*	3	7	*	3	17	*	4	20	*	8	14	293	5	Fortified wine
2806	4164	68	3488	4983	70	2747	3790	72	2382	3934	60	2839	4203	68	Beer & lager†††
238	*	5	188	*	10	309	*	8	71	*	4	196	2768	7	Cider & perry†††
2708	2966	92	4082	4325	94	4793	5089	94	5720	6007	95	4616	4902	94	Tea & water††††
		108			219			253			253			833	Base

Table D3(b)

Comparison of total quantities (grams) of food consumed in seven days in two surveys: 1986/87 Adults Survey; 2000/01 NDNS Adults aged 19 to 64 years: women

Type of food	Women aged (years): 1986/87 Adults Survey**												All women		
	16–24			25–34			35–49			50–64					
	Mean all	Mean consumers	% consumers	Mean all	Mean consumers	% consumers	Mean all	Mean consumers	% consumers	Mean all	Mean consumers	% consumers	Mean all	Mean consumers	% consumers
	g	g	%	g	g	%	g	g	%	g	g	%	g	g	%
Pasta, rice & other miscellaneous cereals	254	334	76	249	319	78	198	282	70	104	184	57	195	281	70
of which:															
Pasta	89	273	33	75	208	36	53	209	26	33	193	17	59	219	27
Rice	79	235	34	92	246	38	84	248	34	39	218	18	73	240	31
Bread	567	567	100	587	592	99	579	583	99	627	632	99	591	595	99
of which:															
White bread	367	390	94	354	398	89	314	372	84	302	370	82	329	381	86
Wholemeal bread	131	298	44	142	286	49	177	303	58	209	341	62	169	310	55
Breakfast cereals	120	186	65	124	205	61	128	229	56	114	205	56	122	209	59
Biscuits, buns, cakes, pastries & fruit pies	224	267	84	248	277	89	347	367	95	342	364	94	302	331	91
of which:															
Biscuits	72	104	70	93	120	78	111	133	83	98	118	83	97	122	80
Fruit pies	12	122	10	16	123	13	32	138	23	38	164	23	26	143	19
Buns, cakes & pastries	140	198	71	138	194	71	205	253	81	206	248	83	179	231	78
Puddings (including dairy desserts & ice cream)	170	292	58	164	262	63	218	309	71	223	309	72	199	296	67
of which:															
Ice cream	37	113	33	34	113	30	45	110	41	42	112	38	40	112	36
Milk****	1277	1349	95	1357	1443	94	1590	1637	97	1480	1540	96	1456	1520	96
of which:															
Whole milk	1053	1206	87	966	1126	86	1042	1176	89	1013	1161	87	1019	1166	87
Semi-skimmed milk	119	702	17	209	744	28	287	1022	28	263	1183	22	234	949	25
Skimmed milk	106	556	19	183	906	20	261	1143	23	204	961	21	202	955	21
Cheese	92	130	71	102	126	81	110	133	82	115	135	85	106	132	81
of which:															
Cottage cheese	12	*	6	10	*	11	12	130	9	17	132	13	13	127	10
Other cheese	80	116	69	92	117	79	98	122	80	98	116	85	94	118	79
Yogurt & fromage frais	104	311	33	98	285	34	100	314	32	110	334	33	103	312	33
Eggs & egg dishes	111	154	72	134	175	76	144	182	79	137	167	82	134	172	78
Fats & oils	92	95	96	115	120	95	106	108	98	117	120	97	108	112	97
of which:															
Butter	33	53	62	44	73	60	42	69	61	51	76	67	43	69	62
Meat & meat products	841	878	96	817	843	97	851	864	98	773	784	99	821	841	98
of which:															
Bacon & ham	67	100	67	74	108	68	87	115	76	95	123	77	83	113	73
Beef, veal & dishes	201	292	69	224	320	70	218	296	74	183	251	73	207	289	72
Lamb & dishes	49	167	29	34	156	22	52	158	33	63	167	38	50	162	31
Pork & dishes	56	135	42	54	130	41	49	127	38	53	133	40	52	131	40
Coated chicken & turkey	19	*	11	13	*	9	11	136	8	6	*	5	11	144	8
Chicken & turkey dishes	122	213	57	129	217	59	151	220	69	127	219	58	135	218	62
Liver, liver products & dishes	21	116	18	21	118	18	32	116	27	33	109	30	28	114	24
Burgers & kebabs	70	164	43	49	156	31	33	127	26	13	102	13	38	142	27
Sausages	53	112	47	58	119	49	51	103	50	50	112	45	53	111	48
Meat pies & pastries	104	219	48	91	186	49	93	201	46	85	190	45	93	198	47
Other meat & meat products	80	209	38	71	149	47	74	172	43	65	140	47	72	163	44

NDNS adults aged 19 to 64, Volume 5 2004

															Type of food
2000/01 NDNS* **												**All women**			
19–24			25–34			35–49			50–64						
Mean all	Mean consumers	% consumers	Mean all	Mean consumers	% consumers	Mean all	Mean consumers	% consumers	Mean all	Mean consumers	% consumers	Mean all	Mean consumers	% consumers	
g	g	%	g	g	%	g	g	%	g	g	%	g	g	%	
520	584	89	512	560	92	446	530	84	317	405	78	433	511	85	Pasta, rice & other miscellaneous cereals
															of which:
270	417	64	198	333	60	169	338	50	123	266	46	174	330	53	Pasta
123	241	51	199	342	58	196	371	53	127	303	42	168	332	51	Rice
591	603	98	569	579	99	573	583	98	544	555	98	566	576	98	Bread
															of which:
438	473	92	353	388	91	353	387	91	323	393	82	354	400	89	White bread
24	*	15	88	249	35	102	238	43	110	236	47	92	236	39	Wholemeal bread
122	224	55	138	202	69	190	269	71	245	325	75	186	267	70	Breakfast cereals
102	156	65	186	222	84	209	242	86	254	282	90	204	242	84	Biscuits, buns, cakes, pastries & fruit pies
															of which:
50	89	56	61	92	66	79	114	69	82	113	73	72	106	68	Biscuits
3	*	3	10	*	9	13	*	9	24	146	17	14	137	11	Fruit pies
49	144	34	114	180	63	117	179	65	148	221	67	117	190	62	Buns, cakes & pastries
123	251	49	112	240	47	131	234	56	166	278	59	135	251	54	Puddings (including dairy desserts & ice cream)
															of which:
48	*	28	38	144	26	35	136	26	46	145	31	40	145	28	Ice cream
1068	1236	87	1137	1196	95	1457	1550	94	1488	1581	94	1345	1440	93	Milk****
															of which:
353	1128	32	322	755	43	326	958	34	242	763	32	304	866	35	Whole milk
516	767	67	670	941	71	850	1150	74	906	1226	74	785	1082	73	Semi-skimmed milk
198	*	15	145	802	18	282	1255	22	340	1290	26	257	1179	22	Skimmed milk
87	132	66	106	133	80	89	122	73	99	125	79	96	127	75	Cheese
															of which:
9	*	6	16	*	10	11	*	5	15	*	9	13	172	8	Cottage cheese
78	125	63	90	116	78	78	110	71	84	109	77	83	113	73	Other cheese
121	387	32	138	326	42	177	400	44	209	456	46	171	399	43	Yogurt & fromage frais
92	195	47	88	151	59	113	168	67	135	178	76	111	170	65	Eggs & egg dishes
55	64	87	60	64	94	69	76	90	75	83	91	67	74	91	Fats & oils
															of which:
10	30	35	15	38	39	19	44	43	27	59	47	19	46	42	Butter
946	1030	92	805	925	87	919	990	93	832	869	96	870	943	92	Meat & meat products
															of which:
62	99	63	73	126	58	74	115	64	86	122	70	76	118	64	Bacon & ham
233	456	51	175	327	54	214	351	61	208	351	59	205	357	58	Beef, veal & dishes
25	*	16	30	184	17	44	246	18	50	176	29	40	197	21	Lamb & dishes
35	*	20	39	148	26	57	189	30	52	185	28	48	178	27	Pork & dishes
78	229	34	44	171	26	48	179	26	24	168	14	43	183	24	Coated chicken & turkey
264	329	80	273	375	73	304	409	74	249	305	81	276	360	77	Chicken & turkey dishes
3	*	4	4	*	3	7	*	8	10	*	10	6	97	7	Liver, liver products & dishes
104	307	34	50	232	22	32	178	18	11	*	8	39	216	18	Burgers & kebabs
56	138	41	48	133	36	43	117	37	37	118	31	44	124	35	Sausages
65	222	29	55	181	30	71	202	35	63	191	33	64	196	33	Meat pies & pastries
22	*	22	14	*	13	25	123	20	44	153	29	27	129	21	Other meat & meat products

Type of food	Women aged (years):												All women		
	1986/87 Adults Survey**														
	16–24			25–34			35–49			50–64					
	Mean all	Mean consum-ers	% consum-ers	Mean all	Mean consum-ers	% consum-ers	Mean all	Mean consum-ers	% consum-ers	Mean all	Mean consum-ers	% consum-ers	Mean all	Mean consum-ers	% consum-ers
	g	g	%	g	g	%	g	g	%	g	g	%	g	g	%
Fish & fish dishes	134	195	69	130	176	74	170	220	77	193	236	82	160	211	76
of which:															
White fish	100	187	53	87	159	55	113	187	60	137	202	68	111	186	60
Oily fish†	26	101	26	31	94	33	43	114	38	47	111	42	39	107	36
Shellfish	8	*	10	12	74	16	14	75	18	9	70	13	11	75	15
Vegetables & vegetable dishes															
(excluding potatoes)	700	704	100	828	831	100	905	910	100	965	968	100	868	872	100
of which:															
Raw carrots	8	*	12	9	62	15	17	80	21	12	71	17	12	72	17
Other raw & salad vegetables	82	122	68	120	172	70	139	176	79	132	172	77	123	166	74
Raw tomatoes	68	117	58	95	141	67	112	150	75	135	171	79	106	150	71
Peas	94	127	74	98	136	72	92	128	72	90	136	66	93	132	71
Green beans	16	80	20	15	87	17	19	92	21	32	121	27	21	98	21
Baked beans	92	178	52	105	200	53	66	159	42	51	146	35	76	171	44
Leafy green vegetables	56	114	49	74	145	51	106	154	69	138	200	69	99	160	62
Carrots - not raw	45	90	50	61	107	57	66	109	61	73	120	61	63	109	58
Tomatoes - not raw	5	*	10	9	67	14	15	75	20	23	92	24	14	77	18
Other vegetables	236	284	83	242	282	86	273	300	91	278	311	89	261	296	88
Potatoes	810	836	97	656	667	98	660	670	98	669	694	97	687	703	98
of which:															
Potato chips	348	436	80	226	317	71	194	282	69	139	236	59	214	311	69
Fried/roast potatoes & fried															
potato products	85	175	49	73	154	47	76	147	52	69	149	46	75	154	49
Potato products, not fried	5	*	4	4	*	3	4	106	4	4	113	4	4	114	4
Other potatoes & potato dishes	371	420	88	354	415	85	385	*	93	457	*	93	394	435	91
Savoury snacks	67	94	71	44	69	63	32	61	52	17	55	30	37	70	52
Fruit (excluding fruit juice)	371	501	74	419	527	79	580	678	86	709	809	88	540	654	83
of which:															
Apples & pears	139	316	44	167	323	52	206	311	66	250	390	64	197	336	59
Citrus fruit	65	261	25	59	235	25	78	251	31	121	297	41	82	265	31
Bananas	49	179	28	67	187	36	77	200	38	83	200	41	72	195	37
Canned fruit in juice	12	*	7	15	*	10	21	229	9	20	173	12	18	184	10
Canned fruit in syrup	19	*	15	15	109	14	25	130	19	30	162	19	23	135	17
Other fruit	88	248	35	96	244	39	173	325	53	206	385	53	149	317	47
Nuts	5	*	7	9	65	14	11	84	14	7	49	14	9	68	13
Sugars, preserves & sweet spreads	118	145	82	123	158	78	143	179	80	93	119	78	121	153	79
of which:															
Table sugar	97	141	69	97	162	60	106	178	60	46	99	47	87	150	58
Preserves	19	52	37	24	53	45	34	64	53	45	78	58	32	64	50
Sweet spreads, fillings & icings	1	*	6	2	*	5	3	29	9	2	*	6	2	30	7
Confectionery	123	169	73	78	115	68	66	107	62	52	98	53	75	119	63
of which:															
Sugar confectionery	20	68	30	10	23	42	8	33	25	11	50	21	11	46	25
Chocolate confectionery	103	147	70	68	63	108	58	104	56	42	88	48	64	111	58
Fruit juice	311	594	52	312	590	53	259	534	49	259	560	46	280	565	50
Soft drinks, not low calorie††	1200	1417	85	697	1019	68	477	832	57	280	605	46	600	972	62
Soft drinks, low calorie††	200	788	25	193	978	20	160	788	20	85	583	15	155	793	20

	2000/01 NDNS***												All women			Type of food
	19–24			25–34			35–49			50–64						
	Mean all	Mean consum-ers	% consum-ers	Mean all	Mean consum-ers	% consum-ers	Mean all	Mean consum-ers	% consum-ers	Mean all	Mean consum-ers	% consum-ers	Mean all	Mean consum-ers	% consum-ers	
	g	g	%	g	g	%	g	g	%	g	g	%	g	g	%	
	144	239	61	151	232	65	215	289	74	298	356	83	216	294	73	Fish & fish dishes
																of which:
	55	175	32	62	164	38	96	208	46	134	226	59	94	204	46	White fish
	68	176	38	63	167	37	86	180	48	126	217	58	90	190	47	Oily fish[†]
	22	*	16	26	131	20	33	144	23	38	181	21	31	151	21	Shellfish
																Vegetables & vegetable dishes
	626	639	98	911	924	99	970	980	99	1004	1006	100	926	935	99	(excluding potatoes)
																of which:
	11	*	12	8	48	17	12	68	19	8	57	15	10	62	16	Raw carrots
	102	141	72	158	188	84	176	214	82	162	203	80	159	197	81	Other raw & salad vegetables
	74	131	57	106	155	69	124	179	69	143	181	79	120	170	70	Raw tomatoes
	46	125	37	46	99	47	64	117	55	68	115	59	59	113	52	Peas
	16	*	20	14	98	15	19	99	19	37	114	33	23	103	22	Green beans
	89	198	45	103	225	46	84	205	41	68	192	35	84	206	41	Baked beans
	41	96	43	55	123	45	82	148	56	126	181	70	84	150	56	Leafy green vegetables
	35	83	42	41	91	45	58	100	58	79	117	68	57	103	56	Carrots - not raw
	13	*	10	33	136	24	28	125	22	27	96	28	27	118	23	Tomatoes - not raw
	199	246	81	347	424	82	322	371	87	287	329	87	304	357	85	Other vegetables
	761	788	97	599	618	97	636	656	97	670	695	96	652	674	97	Potatoes
																of which:
	327	434	76	217	302	72	180	271	66	152	247	62	198	294	67	Potato chips
																Fried/roast potatoes & fried
	72	166	43	60	155	39	76	179	42	78	179	44	72	172	42	potato products
	9	*	8	2	*	4	4	*	5	7	*	4	5	115	5	Potato products, not fried
	353	455	78	320	415	77	375	431	87	433	494	88	376	449	84	Other potatoes & potato dishes
	83	108	76	64	92	69	41	73	57	20	51	39	45	80	57	Savoury snacks
	379	552	69	521	648	80	687	853	81	1060	1141	93	720	871	83	Fruit (excluding fruit juice)
																of which:
	113	283	40	183	365	50	188	348	54	294	482	61	209	390	54	Apples & pears
	47	*	22	66	301	22	100	326	31	146	363	40	99	327	30	Citrus fruit
	81	291	28	156	300	52	194	344	56	260	379	69	191	344	56	Bananas
	4	*	3	9	*	7	12	*	7	24	176	14	14	169	8	Canned fruit in juice
	6	*	2	3	*	3	5	*	4	19	*	10	8	165	5	Canned fruit in syrup
	127	306	41	103	256	40	188	362	52	318	502	63	199	387	51	Other fruit
	11	66	17	10	54	19	13	69	19	13	58	23	12	62	20	Nuts
	52	85	61	75	109	69	87	122	71	83	122	68	79	115	68	Sugars, preserves & sweet spreads
																of which:
	41	90	45	51	103	50	63	129	48	56	118	47	55	115	48	Table sugar
	8	*	21	22	60	36	21	52	41	26	57	45	21	55	39	Preserves
	3	*	11	2	*	7	3	*	8	1	*	5	2	29	7	Sweet spreads, fillings & icings
	89	140	63	77	114	68	80	117	68	66	115	57	76	118	64	Confectionery
																of which:
	19	61	31	12	49	24	14	54	27	19	89	21	16	63	25	Sugar confectionery
	70	118	60	65	111	58	65	106	62	47	94	50	60	106	57	Chocolate confectionery
	353	701	50	316	625	50	301	690	44	358	766	47	327	697	47	Fruit juice
	1705	2179	78	771	1230	63	560	1041	54	416	940	44	702	1254	56	Soft drinks, not low calorie[††]
	1002	1889	53	1185	2054	58	555	1449	38	379	1190	32	705	1650	43	Soft drinks, low calorie[††]

Type of food	Women aged (years):														
	1986/87 Adults Survey**												All women		
	16–24			25–34			35–49			50–64					
	Mean all	Mean consum-ers	% consum-ers	Mean all	Mean consum-ers	% consum-ers	Mean all	Mean consum-ers	% consum-ers	Mean all	Mean consum-ers	% consum-ers	Mean all	Mean consum-ers	% consum-ers
	g	g	%	g	g	%	g	g	%	g	g	%	g	g	%
Alcoholic drinks	683	1331	51	747	1092	68	633	994	64	405	704	58	609	997	61
of which:															
Liqueurs	10	*	11	5	*	8	4	*	5	4	*	6	5	76	7
Spirits	18	116	16	21	91	23	26	117	22	24	115	21	23	110	21
Wine†††	131	527	25	206	505	41	223	526	42	105	355	30	173	485	36
Fortified wine	18	*	15	33	181	18	41	219	19	45	175	25	36	184	20
Beer & lager†††	326	1709	19	386	1220	32	304	1410	22	204	1201	17	301	1352	22
Cider & perry†††	181	*	13	96	*	11	34	*	7	24	*	6	71	836	9
Tea & water††††	3991	3991	100	5817	5840	100	6717	6717	100	6631	6631	100	6026	6031	100
Base			189			253			385			283			1110

* Numbers of consumers too small to calculate mean/standard deviation values reliably.

** Gregory JR et al. The Dietary and Nutritional Survey of British Adults. HMSO (London, 1990)
Food consumption data from the 1986/87 Adults Survey has been recalculated, and the data for both surveys restructured into specific food groups to allow comparisons to be made. Consequently, there may be small discrepancies between the 1986/87 data as published in 1990 and that presented in this volume.

*** Data shown in this table may differ from data presented in Tables 2.10(a) and 2.11(a) of Volume 1 due to an error in the application of the dilution factor. Revised Volume 1 tables are available online at www.food.gov.uk.

**** Includes whole milk, semi-skimmed milk and skimmed milk only. Other milks and creams excluded as data are not comparable between the two surveys due to differences in the dietary recording methodology.

† Oily fish includes canned tuna.

†† Figures for soft drinks, low calorie and not low calorie, are as consumed, that is includes concentrated drinks plus diluent.

††† Includes low-alcohol variations.

†††† Water includes tap water, and bottled water without added sugar or artificial sweeteners; coffee is excluded from this table as data between the two surveys on consumption of coffee are not comparable due to differences in dietary recording methodology.

															Type of food
2000/01 NDNS* **												**All women**			
19–24			25–34			35–49			50–64						
Mean all	Mean consum-ers	% consum-ers	Mean all	Mean consum-ers	% consum-ers	Mean all	Mean consum-ers	% consum-ers	Mean all	Mean consum-ers	% consum-ers	Mean all	Mean consum-ers	% consum-ers	
g	g	%	g	g	%	g	g	%	g	g	%	g	g	%	
1552	2194	71	1069	1554	69	960	1428	67	678	1041	65	973	1444	67	Alcoholic drinks
															of which:
6	*	10	7	*	8	6	*	8	3	*	6	5	72	8	Liqueurs
32	*	27	20	116	18	27	139	19	37	162	23	29	139	21	Spirits
239	627	38	326	720	45	349	754	46	412	839	49	349	760	46	Wine[†††]
4	*	3	16	*	6	18	*	9	22	*	11	17	216	8	Fortified wine
864	2593	34	555	1619	34	413	1596	26	163	1099	15	427	1671	25	Beer & lager[†††]
69	*	2	49	*	3	65	*	3	19	*	4	48	*	3	Cider & perry[†††]
3250	3437	95	4844	4952	98	5491	5815	94	6049	6487	93	5238	5519	95	Tea & water[††††]
		104			210			318			259			891	Base

Table D3(c)

Comparison of total quantities (grams) of food consumed in seven days in two surveys: 1986/87 Adults Survey; 2000/01 NDNS Adults aged 19 to 64 years: all

Type of food	All					
	1986/87 Adults Survey**			2000/01 NDNS***		
	Mean all	Mean consumers	% consumers	Mean all	Mean consumers	% consumers
	g	g	%	g	g	%
Pasta, rice & other miscellaneous cereals	236	334	71	507	585	87
of which:						
Pasta	63	245	26	193	366	53
Rice	99	300	33	196	376	52
Bread	761	766	100	706	716	99
of which:						
White bread	458	524	87	462	510	91
Wholemeal bread	209	405	52	109	300	36
Breakfast cereals	143	248	58	203	304	67
Biscuits, buns, cakes, pastries & fruit pies	327	363	90	231	277	84
of which:						
Biscuits	100	131	77	83	126	66
Fruit pies	34	163	21	19	153	12
Buns, cakes & pastries	193	257	75	130	216	60
Puddings (including dairy desserts & ice cream)	228	343	66	142	276	51
of which:						
Ice cream	45	129	35	42	155	27
Milk****	1583	1648	96	1430	1522	94
of which:						
Whole milk	1148	1303	88	337	947	36
Semi-skimmed milk	255	1119	23	877	1198	73
Skimmed milk	181	989	18	215	1176	18
Cheese	120	148	81	106	138	77
of which:						
Cottage cheese	8	120	7	9	168	5
Other cheese	111	140	80	98	129	76
Yogurt & fromage frais	81	303	27	153	401	38
Eggs & egg dishes	160	200	80	133	197	68
Fats & oils	130	134	97	86	93	93
of which:						
Butter	47	78	60	22	54	41
Meat, meat dishes & meat products	1049	1066	98	1125	1186	95
of which:						
Bacon & ham	109	142	77	105	149	71
Beef, veal & dishes	257	340	76	249	399	62
Lamb & dishes	61	191	32	51	226	22
Pork & dishes	67	160	42	63	207	30
Coated chicken & turkey	13	156	8	48	195	24
Chicken & turkey dishes	159	247	64	326	411	79
Liver, liver products & dishes	29	120	24	11	119	9
Burgers & kebabs	50	171	29	61	244	25
Sausages	75	142	53	68	151	45
Meat pies & pastries	134	253	53	101	256	39
Other meat & meat products	95	201	47	43	164	26

Type of food	All					
	1986/87 Adults Survey**			**2000/01 NDNS*****		
	Mean all	Mean consumers	% consumers	Mean all	Mean consumers	% consumers
	g	g	%	g	g	%
Fish & fish dishes	186	245	76	217	304	71
of which:						
White fish	126	206	61	104	221	47
Oily fish†	47	135	35	86	194	44
Shellfish	13	98	14	28	144	19
Vegetables & vegetable dishes (excluding potatoes)	956	961	100	943	952	99
of which:						
Raw carrots	11	72	15	10	69	14
Other raw & salad vegetables	120	166	72	144	184	78
Raw tomatoes	107	155	69	113	165	69
Peas	111	155	72	73	132	55
Green beans	24	111	22	23	108	22
Baked beans	101	213	48	113	255	44
Leafy green vegetables	110	178	62	80	152	53
Carrots - not raw	72	120	60	59	106	56
Tomatoes - not raw	18	90	20	32	131	24
Other vegetables	284	322	88	295	349	84
Potatoes	883	900	98	734	753	97
of which:						
Potato chips	291	389	75	248	348	71
Fried/roast potatoes & fried potato products	102	197	52	85	203	42
Potato products, not fried	4	115	4	9	146	6
Other potatoes & potato dishes	486	537	90	391	469	84
Savoury snacks	41	81	51	52	92	56
Fruit (excluding fruit juice)	501	638	79	666	841	79
of which:						
Apples & pears	195	356	55	212	412	51
Citrus fruit	71	258	28	87	315	28
Bananas	64	201	32	184	352	52
Canned fruit in juice	15	167	9	15	176	8
Canned fruit in syrup	27	152	18	11	201	5
Other fruit	129	306	42	157	353	44
Nuts	8	64	12	15	71	20
Sugars, preserves & sweet spreads	164	199	82	106	147	72
of which:						
Table sugar	126	193	65	80	148	54
Preserves	37	76	48	24	64	37
Sweet spreads, fillings & icings	2	29	6	2	32	7
Confectionery	74	124	59	82	131	62
of which:						
Sugar confectionery	10	50	21	15	67	23
Chocolate confectionery	63	118	54	66	119	56
Fruit juice	269	606	44	333	742	45
Soft drinks, not low calorie††	677	1103	61	882	1474	60
Soft drinks, low calorie††	131	844	16	653	1680	39

Type of food	All					
	1986/87 Adults Survey**			2000/01 NDNS***		
	Mean all	Mean consumers	% consumers	Mean all	Mean consumers	% consumers
	g	g	%	g	g	%
Alcoholic drinks	2116	3083	69	2193	2974	74
of which:						
Liqueurs	3	72	5	4	82	5
Spirits	32	145	22	34	166	20
Wine†††	172	520	33	341	825	41
Fortified wine	31	211	15	16	244	6
Beer & lager†††	1785	4155	43	1592	3474	46
Cider & perry†††	92	1007	9	119	2353	5
Tea & water††††	6047	6080	100	4937	5222	95
Base			2197			1724

*	Numbers of consumers too small to calculate mean/standard deviation values reliably.
**	Gregory JR et al. The Dietary and Nutritional Survey of British Adults. HMSO (London, 1990).
	Food consumption data from the 1986/87 Adults Survey has been recalculated, and the data for both surveys restructured into specific food groups to allow comparisons to be made. Consequently, there may be small discrepancies between the 1986/87 data as published in 1990 and that presented in this volume.
***	Data shown in this table may differ from data presented in Table 2.14 of Volume 1 due to an error in the application of the dilution factor. Revised Volume 1 tables are available online at www.food.gov.uk.
****	Includes whole milk, semi-skimmed milk and skimmed milk only. Other milks and creams excluded as data are not comparable between the two surveys due to differences in the dietary recording methodology.
†	Oily fish includes canned tuna.
††	Figures for soft drinks, low calorie and not low calorie, are as consumed, that is includes concentrated drinks plus diluent.
†††	Includes low-alcohol variations.
††††	Water includes tap water, and bottled water without added sugar or artificial sweeteners; coffee is excluded from this table as data between the two surveys on consumption of coffee are not comparable due to differences in dietary recording methodology.

Table D4(a):

Main differences in the eating behaviour of respondents in 1986/87 Adults Survey and those in the 2000/01 NDNS: men by age group

Foods more likely to be eaten by men in 1986/87 Adults Survey (compared with men in 2000/01 NDNS):

16–24 years		25–34 years		35–49 years	
Food category	Food type	Food category	Food type	Food category	Food type
	Wholemeal bread		Wholemeal bread		Wholemeal bread
	Fruit pies				
			Biscuits	Biscuits, buns, cakes,	Fruit pies
Puddings (including dairy			Buns, cakes & pastries	pastries & fruit pies	Buns, cakes & pastries
desserts & ice cream)					
	Whole milk	Puddings (including dairy		Puddings (including dairy	
		desserts & ice cream)		desserts & ice cream)	
Eggs & egg dishes			Whole milk		Whole milk
	Pork & dishes		Butter	Eggs & egg dishes	
	Meat pies & pastries		Liver, liver products &	Fats & oils	Butter
	Peas		dishes		Beef, veal & dishes
			Other meat & meat		Lamb & dishes
	Canned fruit in syrup		products		Liver, liver products &
			White fish		dishes
					Other meat & meat
			Peas		products
			Leafy green vegetables		
					White fish
			Canned fruit in syrup		Fried/roast potatoes &
		Sugars, preserves &	Preserves		fried potato products
		sweet spreads			Other potatoes & potato
					dishes
					Canned fruit in syrup
				Sugars, preserves &	Table sugar
				sweet spreads	Preserves
					Fortified wine
				Tea & water**	
Pasta, rice & other	Pasta	Pasta, rice & other	Pasta	Pasta, rice & other	Pasta
miscellaneous cereals	Rice	miscellaneous cereals		miscellaneous cereals	Rice
	Semi-skimmed milk		Semi-skimmed milk	Breakfast cereals	
					Semi-skimmed milk
	Coated chicken & turkey		Coated chicken & turkey	Yogurt & fromage frais	
					Coated chicken & turkey
Soft drinks, not low calorie			Bananas		Chicken & turkey dishes
Soft drinks, low calorie					
			Soft drinks, low calorie		Bananas
				Nuts	
				Confectionery	Chocolate confectionery
				Soft drinks, low calorie	

*   Oily fish includes canned tuna.
** Water includes tap water and bottled water without added sugar or artificial sweeteners.

NDNS adults aged 19 to 64, Volume 5 2004

50–64 years		All men	
Food category	Food type	Food category	Food type
	Buns, cakes & pastries		Wholemeal bread
Puddings (including dairy desserts & ice cream)		Biscuits, buns, cakes, pastries & fruit pies	Biscuits
	Whole milk		Fruit pies
			Buns, cakes & pastries
	Butter	Puddings (including dairy desserts & ice cream)	Ice cream
	Beef, veal & dishes		
	Liver, liver products & dishes		Whole milk
	Other meat & meat products		
	Canned fruit in syrup	Eggs & egg dishes	
	Table sugar		Butter
	Fortified wine		Beef, veal & dishes
			Lamb & dishes
Tea & water**			Pork & dishes
			Meat pies & pastries
			Other meat & meat products
			White fish
			Peas
			Leafy green vegetables
			Fried/roast potatoes & fried potato products
			Other potatoes & potato dishes
			Canned fruit in syrup
		Sugars, preserves & sweet spreads	Table sugar
			Preserves
			Fortified wine
		Tea & water**	
Pasta, rice & other miscellaneous cereals	Pasta	Pasta, rice & other miscellaneous cereals	Pasta
	Rice		Rice
	Semi-skimmed milk		White bread
Yogurt & fromage frais		Breakfast cereals	
	Coated chicken & turkey		Semi-skimmed milk
	Chicken & turkey dishes	Yogurt & fromage frais	
	Bananas		Coated chicken & turkey
			Chicken & turkey dishes
Fruit juice			Oily fish*
Soft drinks, low calorie			Shellfish
			Other raw & salad vegetables
			Potato products, not fried
			Bananas
		Nuts	
		Soft drinks, low calorie	

107

Table D4(b)

Main differences in the eating behaviour of respondents in 1986/87 Adults Survey and those in the 2000/01 NDNS: women by age group

Foods more likely to be eaten by women in 1986/87 Adults Survey (compared with women in 2000/01 NDNS):

16–24 years		25–34 years		35–49 years	
Food category	Food type	Food category	Food type	Food category	Food type
	Wholemeal bread		Wholemeal bread		Wholemeal bread
		Puddings (including dairy desserts & ice cream)		Breakfast cereals	
Biscuits, buns, cakes, pastries & fruit pies	Buns, cakes & pastries			Biscuits, buns, cakes, pastries & fruit pies	Biscuits
	Whole milk		Whole milk		Fruit pies
					Buns, cakes & pastries
Eggs & egg dishes		Eggs & egg dishes		Puddings (including dairy desserts & ice cream)	Ice cream
	Butter		Butter		
					Whole milk
	Pork & dishes	Meat & meat products	Beef, veal & dishes	Cheese	Other cheese
	Liver, liver products & dishes		Pork & dishes		
	Meat pies & pastries		Liver, liver products & dishes	Eggs & egg dishes	
	White fish		Meat pies & pastries	Fats & oils	Butter
			Other meat & meat products	Meat & meat products	Bacon & ham
	Peas		White fish		Beef, veal & dishes
					Lamb & dishes
	Canned fruit in syrup				Liver, liver products & dishes
Sugars, preserves & sweet spreads	Table sugar		Peas		Sausages
					Meat pies & pastries
			Canned fruit in syrup		Other meat & meat products
	Fortified wine				
	Cider & perry		Sugar confectionery		White fish
			Fortified wine		Peas
			Cider & perry		Leafy green vegetables
					Apples & pears
					Canned fruit in syrup
					Table sugar
					Preserves
					Fortified wine
				Tea & water**	
	Pasta	Pasta, rice & other miscellaneous cereals	Pasta	Pasta, rice & other miscellaneous cereals	Pasta
			Rice		Rice
	Semi-skimmed milk		Semi-skimmed milk		Semi-skimmed milk
	Coated chicken & turkey			Yogurt & fromage frais	
	Chicken & turkey dishes		Coated chicken & turkey		Coated chicken & turkey
			Chicken & turkey dishes		
Soft drinks, low calorie			Other raw & salad vegetables		Bananas
Alcoholic drinks				Soft drinks, low calorie	
			Bananas		
		Soft drinks, low calorie			

*   Oily fish includes canned tuna.
**   Water includes tap water and bottled water without added sugar or artificial sweeteners.
*** Includes low alcohol variations.

50–64 years		All women	
Food category	Food type	Food category	Food type
	Wholemeal bread		Wholemeal bread
	Buns, cakes & pastries	Biscuits, buns, cakes, pastries & fruit pies	Biscuits
			Fruit pies
			Buns, cakes & pastries
Puddings (including dairy desserts & ice cream)		Puddings (including dairy desserts & ice cream)	Ice cream
	Whole milk		Whole milk
Fats & oils	Butter		
	Beef, veal & dishes	Cheese	Other cheese
	Pork & dishes		
	Liver, liver products & dishes	Eggs & egg dishes	
	Sausages		
	Meat pies & pastries	Fats & oils	Butter
	Other meat & meat products		
	Canned fruit in syrup	Meat & meat products	Bacon & ham
			Beef, veal & dishes
	Preserves		Lamb & dishes
	Fortified wine		Liver, liver products & dishes
			Burgers & kebabs
Tea & water**			Sausages
			Meat pies & pastries
			Other meat & meat products
			White fish
			Peas
			Fried/roast potatoes & fried potato products
			Other potatoes & potato dishes
			Canned fruit in syrup
		Sugars, preserves & sweet spreads	Table sugar
			Preserves
			Fortified wine
			Cider & perry
		Tea & water**	
Pasta, rice & other miscellaneous cereals	Pasta	Pasta, rice & other miscellaneous cereals	Pasta
	Rice		Rice
Breakfast cereals		Breakfast cereals	
	Semi-skimmed milk		Semi-skimmed milk
Yogurt & fromage frais		Yogurt & fromage frais	
	Coated chicken & turkey		Coated chicken & turkey
	Chicken & turkey dishes		Chicken & turkey dishes
	Oily fish*		Oily fish*
			Shellfish
	Bananas		Other raw & salad vegetables
Soft drinks, low calorie			Bananas
	Wine***	Nuts	
		Soft drinks, low calorie	
		Alcoholic drinks	Wine***

Table D5:

Main differences in the total quantity of foods consumed by respondents in 1986/87 Adults Survey and those in the 2000/01 NDNS: all respondents, including non-consumers

Greater quantity eaten by respondents in:

1986/87 Adults Survey (compared with 2000/01 NDNS)		2000/01 NDNS (compared with 1986/87 Adults Survey)	
Food category	Food type	Food category	Food type
Bread	Wholemeal bread	Pasta, rice & other miscellaneous cereals	Pasta
			Rice
Biscuits, buns, cakes, pastries & fruit pies	Biscuits		
	Fruit pies	Breakfast cereals	
	Buns, cakes & pastries		Semi-skimmed milk
Puddings (including dairy desserts & ice cream)		Yogurt & fromage frais	
Milk**	Whole milk	Meat & meat products	Coated chicken & turkey
			Chicken & turkey dishes
			Burgers & kebabs
Cheese	Other cheese	Fish & fish dishes	Oily fish*
Eggs & egg dishes			Shellfish
Fats & oils	Butter		Other raw & salad vegetables
			Tomatoes - not raw
	Liver, liver products & dishes		
	Meat pies & pastries		Potato products - not fried
	Other meat & meat products		
		Savoury snacks	
	White fish		
		Fruit (excluding fruit juice)	Bananas
	Peas		
	Leafy green vegetables	Nuts	
	Carrots - not raw		
		Fruit juice	
Potatoes	Potato chips	Soft drinks, not low calorie	
	Fried/roast potatoes & fried potato products	Soft drinks, low calorie	
	Other potatoes & potato dishes		Wine***
	Canned fruit in syrup		
Sugars, preserves & sweet spreads	Table sugar		
	Preserves		
	Fortified wine		
Tea & water****			

---

*   *Oily fish includes canned tuna.*

**   *Includes whole milk, semi-skimmed and skimmed milk only. Other milks and creams excluded as data are not comparable between the two surveys due to differences in the dietary recording methodology.*

***   *Includes low alcohol variations.*

****   *Water includes tap water and bottled water without added sugar or artificial sweeteners.*

Table D6(a)

Main differences in the total quantities of foods consumed by respondents in 1986/87 Adults Survey and those in the 2000/01 NDNS: men by age group, including non-consumers

Greater quantity eaten by men in 1986/87 Adults Survey (compared with men in 2000/01 NDNS):

16–24 years		25–34 years		35–49 years	
Food category	Food type	Food category	Food type	Food category	Food type
Bread	Wholemeal bread		Wholemeal bread		Wholemeal bread
Biscuits, buns, cakes, pastries & fruit pies	Fruit pies	Biscuits, buns, cakes, pastries & fruit pies		Biscuits, buns, cakes, pastries & fruit pies	Fruit pies / Buns, cakes & pastries
Puddings (including dairy desserts & ice cream)		Puddings (including dairy desserts & ice cream)	Ice cream	Puddings (including dairy desserts & ice cream)	
Milk*	Whole milk		Whole milk		Whole milk
	Meat pies & pastries / Other meat & meat products	Fats & oils	Butter		Other cheese
			Liver, liver products & dishes	Eggs & egg dishes	
	Peas		Meat pies & pastries	Fats & oils	Butter
	Leafy green vegetables		White fish		Liver, liver products & dishes
Potatoes	Other potatoes & potato dishes		Peas		Other meat & meat products
			Leafy green vegetables		White fish
		Potatoes	Other potatoes & potato dishes		Peas
Sugars, preserves & sweet spreads	Table sugar		Canned fruit in syrup		Leafy green vegetables / Carrots - not raw
Tea & water**		Sugars, preserves & sweet spreads	Preserves	Potatoes	Fried/roast potatoes & fried potato products / Other potatoes & potato dishes
		Tea & water**			Canned fruit in syrup
				Sugars, preserves & sweet spreads	Table sugar / Preserves
					Fortified wine
				Tea & water**	

50–64 years		All men	
Food category	Food type	Food category	Food type
	Wholemeal bread	Bread	Wholemeal bread
Puddings (including dairy desserts & ice cream)		Biscuits, buns, cakes, pastries & fruit pies	Fruit pies Buns, cakes & pastries
	Whole milk	Puddings (including dairy desserts & ice cream)	
Fats & oils	Butter	Milk	Whole milk
	Leafy green vegetables	Eggs & egg dishes	
Potatoes	Other potatoes & potato dishes	Fats & oils	Butter
Sugars, preserves & sweet spreads	Table sugar		Liver, liver products & dishes Meat pies & pastries Other meat & meat products
Tea & water**			White fish
		Vegetables	Peas Leafy green vegetables Carrots - not raw
		Potatoes	Potato chips Fried/roast potatoes & fried potato products Other potatoes & potato dishes
			Canned fruit in syrup
		Sugars, preserves & sweet spreads	Table sugar Preserves
		Tea & water**	

Greater quantity eaten by men in 2000/01 NDNS (compared with men in 1986/87 Adults Survey):

16–24 years		25–34 years		35–49 years	
Food category	Food type	Food category	Food type	Food category	Food type
Pasta, rice & other miscellaneous cereals	Pasta	Pasta, rice & other miscellaneous cereals	Pasta Rice	Pasta, rice & other miscellaneous cereals	Pasta Rice
	Semi-skimmed milk		Semi-skimmed milk		Semi-skimmed milk
	Coated chicken & turkey Chicken & turkey dishes		Coated chicken & turkey Chicken & turkey dishes	Yogurt & fromage frais	
Soft drinks, not low calorie			Bananas	Meat & meat products	Coated chicken & turkey Chicken & turkey dishes Burgers & kebabs
		Soft drinks, not low calorie Soft drinks, low calorie			Oily fish***
					Tomatoes - not raw
				Savoury snacks	
				Fruit (excluding fruit juice)	Bananas
				Nuts	
				Confectionery	Chocolate confectionery
				Fruit juice Soft drinks, low calorie	
					Wine****

*   *Includes whole milk, semi-skimmed and skimmed milk only. Other milks and creams excluded as data are not comparable between the two surveys due to differences in the dietary recording methodology.*
**   *Water includes tap water and bottled water without added sugar or artificial sweeteners.*
***   *Oily fish includes canned tuna.*
****   *Includes low alcohol variations.*

50–64 years		All men	
Food category	Food type	Food category	Food type
Pasta, rice & other	Pasta	Pasta, rice & other	Pasta
miscellaneous cereals	Rice	miscellaneous cereals	Rice
Breakfast cereals		Breakfast cereals	
	Semi-skimmed milk		Semi-skimmed milk
Yogurt & fromage frais		Yogurt & fromage frais	
	Coated chicken & turkey	Meat & meat products	Coated chicken & turkey
	Chicken & turkey dishes		Chicken & turkey dishes
Fruit (excluding fruit juice)	Bananas		Burgers & kebabs
Fruit juice			Oily fish***
Soft drinks, low calorie			Tomatoes - not raw
	Wine****		Potato products - not fried
		Savoury snacks	
		Fruit (excluding fruit juice)	Bananas
		Nuts	
		Fruit juice	
		Soft drinks, not low calorie	
		Soft drinks, low calorie	
		Wine****	

Table D6(b)

Main differences in the total quantities of foods consumed by respondents in 1986/87 Adults Survey and those in the 2000/01 NDNS: women by age group, including non-consumers

Greater quantity eaten by women in 1986/87 Adults Survey (compared with women in 2000/01 NDNS):

16–24 years		25–34 years		35–49 years	
Food category	Food type	Food category	Food type	Food category	Food type
	Wholemeal bread		Wholemeal bread		Wholemeal bread
Biscuits, buns, cakes, pastries & fruit pies	Buns, cakes & pastries	Biscuits, buns, cakes, pastries & fruit pies	Biscuits	Biscuits, buns, cakes, pastries & fruit pies	Biscuits
					Fruit pies
					Buns, cakes & pastries
	Whole milk		Whole milk		
				Puddings (including dairy desserts & ice cream)	
Fats & oils	Butter		Eggs & egg dishes		
					Whole milk
	Liver, liver products & dishes	Fats & oils	Butter		
	Other meat & meat products				
					Other cheese
			Liver, liver products & dishes		
	White fish		Meat pies & pastries		Eggs & egg dishes
Sugars, preserves & sweet spreads	Table sugar		Other meat & meat products	Fats & oils	Butter
					Liver, liver products & dishes
			White fish		Other meat & meat products
			Peas		Peas
			Canned fruit in syrup		Canned fruit in syrup
		Sugars, preserves & sweet spreads	Table sugar	Sugars, preserves & sweet spreads	Table sugar
					Preserves
			Tea & water*		Tea & water*

50–64 years		All women	
Food category	Food type	Food category	Food type
Bread	Wholemeal bread		Wholemeal bread
Biscuits, buns, cakes, pastries & fruit pies	Buns, cakes & pastries	Biscuits, buns, cakes, pastries & fruit pies	Biscuits
			Fruit pies
			Buns, cakes & pastries
Puddings (including dairy desserts & ice cream)		Puddings (including dairy desserts & ice cream)	
	Whole milk		Whole milk
Fats & oils	Butter	Eggs & egg dishes	
	Liver, liver products & dishes		
	Preserves	Fats & oils	Butter
			Liver, liver products & dishes
			Meat pies & pastries
			Other meat & meat products
			White fish
			Peas
			Canned fruit in syrup
		Sugars, preserves & sweet spreads	Table sugar
			Preserves
			Fortified wine
		Tea & water*	

Greater quantity eaten by women in 2000/01 NDNS (compared with women in 1986/87 Adults Survey):

16–24 years		25–34 years		35–49 years	
Food category	Food type	Food category	Food type	Food category	Food type
Pasta, rice & other miscellaneous cereals	Pasta	Pasta, rice & other miscellaneous cereals	Pasta	Pasta, rice & other miscellaneous cereals	Pasta
			Rice		Rice
	Semi-skimmed milk		Semi-skimmed milk	Breakfast cereals	
	Coated chicken & turkey		Coated chicken & turkey		Semi-skimmed milk
	Chicken & turkey dishes		Chicken & turkey dishes		
				Yogurt & fromage frais	
Soft drinks, low calorie			Oily fish		
Alcoholic drinks					Coated chicken & turkey
			Tomatoes - not raw		Chicken & turkey dishes
			Other vegetables		
					Oily fish**
		Savoury snacks			Shellfish
			Bananas		Bananas
		Soft drinks, low calorie		Soft drinks, low calorie	
				Alcoholic drinks	Wine***

*   Water includes tap water and bottled water without added sugar or artificial sweeteners.
**   Oily fish includes canned tuna.
***   Includes low alcohol variations.

NDNS adults aged 19 to 64, Volume 5 2004

50–64 years		All women	
Food category	Food type	Food category	Food type
Pasta, rice & other miscellaneous cereals	Pasta Rice	Pasta, rice & other miscellaneous cereals	Pasta Rice
Breakfast cereals		Breakfast cereals	
	Semi-skimmed milk		Semi-skimmed milk
Yogurt & fromage frais		Yogurt & fromage frais	
	Coated chicken & turkey Chicken & turkey dishes		Coated chicken & turkey Chicken & turkey dishes
Fish & fish dishes	Oily fish** Shellfish	Fish & fish dishes	Oily fish** Shellfish
Fruit (excluding fruit juice)	Bananas Other fruit		Other raw & salad vegetables Tomatoes - not raw
Soft drinks, low calorie		Savoury snacks	
Alcoholic drinks	Wine***	Fruit (excluding fruit juice)	Bananas Other fruit
		Soft drinks, low calorie	
		Alcoholic drinks	Wine***

Appendix E Weights for results from analysis of blood samples

Weights were derived for results from the analysis of blood samples (see Appendix B). Three weighting factors were calculated based on similar numbers of reported results for different analytes and similarity of socio-demographic characteristics. These are shown below for the blood analytes discussed in this Volume. For the complete listing see Appendix C, Volume 4[1].

The three groups were as follows:

Group 1: Non-response weight based on number of haemoglobin results

Applies to:

Haemoglobin
Serum ferritin
Plasma vitamin C
Red cell folate
Serum folate
Serum vitamin B_{12}
Erythrocyte Transketolase Activation Coefficient (ETKAC)
Erythrocyte Glutathione Reductase Activation Coefficient (EGRAC)
Erythrocyte Aspartate Aminotransferase Activation Coefficient (EAATAC)

Group 2: Non-response weight based on number of results for plasma iron

Applies to:

Plasma iron % saturation
Plasma 25-hydroxyvitamin D (25-OHD)
Plasma α-tocopherol to total cholesterol ratio
Plasma total cholesterol

Group 3: Non-response weight based on number of plasma retinol results

Applies to:

Plasma retinol

References and endnotes

[1] Ruston D, Hoare J, Henderson L, Gregory J, Bates CJ, Prentice A, Birch M, Swan G, Farron M. *National Diet and Nutrition Survey: adults aged 19 to 64 years. Volume 4: Nutritional status (anthropometry and blood analytes), blood pressure and physical activity.* TSO (London, 2004).

Appendix F Glossary of abbreviations, terms and survey definitions

Base	Number of cases within a cell or group. Bases included in this report are *weighted* (*see* Appendix B).
Benefits (receiving)	Receipt of Working Families Tax Credit by the respondent or anyone in their household at the time of the interview, or receipt of Income Support, or (Income related) Job Seeker's Allowance by the respondent or anyone in their household in the 14 days prior to the date of interview.
BMI	*See* Body Mass Index
Body Mass Index	A measure of body 'fatness' which standardises weight for height: calculated as [weight(kg)/height(m^2)]. Also known as the Quetelet Index.
COMA	The Committee on Medical Aspects of Food and Nutrition Policy.
CAPI	Computer assisted personal interviewing.
Deft	Design factor; see Notes to Tables and Appendix C.
DH	The Department of Health.
Diary sample	Respondents for whom a seven-day dietary record was obtained.
DNA	Deoxyribonucleic acid. DNA molecules carry the genetic information necessary for the organisation and functioning of most living cells.
Dna	does not apply.
Doubly labelled water (DLW)	A method for assessing total energy expenditure, used to validate dietary assessment methods by comparison with esimated energy intake. The respondent drinks a measured dose of water labelled with the stable isotopes $^2H_2$ and ^{18}O and collects urine samples over the next 10 to 15 days. Energy expenditure is calculated from the excretion rates of the isotopes.
DRV	Dietary Reference Value. The term used to cover LRNI, EAR, RNI and safe intake. (*See* Department of Health. Report on Health and Social Subjects: **41**. *Dietary Reference Values for Food Energy and Nutrients for the United Kingdom*. HMSO (London, 1991)).
EAR	The Estimated Average Requirement of a group of people for energy or protein or a vitamin or mineral. About half will usually need more than the EAR, and half less.
EFS	Expenditure and Food Survey. The National Food Survey was replaced by the Expenditure and Food Survey from 1 April 2001.
Eligible sample	Includes respondents who were aged between 19 and 64 years and not pregnant or breastfeeding.
Extrinsic sugars	Any sugar which is not contained within the cell structure of a food. Examples are sugars in honey, table sugar and lactose in milk and milk products.
HNR	Medical Research Council Human Nutrition Research, Cambridge.
Household	The standard definition used in most surveys carried out by ONS and

	comparable with the 1991 Census definition of a household was used in this survey. A household is defined as a single person or group of people who have the accommodation as their only or main residence and who either share one main meal a day or share the living accommodation. (*See* McCrossan E. *A Handbook for interviewers*. HMSO (London,1991)).
HRP	Household Reference Person. This is the member of the household in whose name the accommodation is owned or rented, or is otherwise responsible for the accommodation. In households with a *sole* householder that person is the household reference person, in households with *joint* householders the person with the *highest income* is taken as the household reference person, if both householders have exactly the same income, the *older* is taken as the household reference person. This differs from Head of Household in that female householders with the highest income are now taken as the HRP, and in the case of joint householders, income then age, rather than sex then age is used to define the HRP.
HSfE	Health Survey for England.
Intrinsic sugars	Any sugar which is contained within the cell structure of a food. Examples are sugars found in fresh fruit which has not been processed.
lc	low calorie.
LRNI	The Lower Reference Nutrient Intake for protein or a vitamin or mineral. An amount of nutrient that is enough for only the few people in the group who have low needs.
MAFF	The Ministry of Agriculture, Fisheries and Food.
Mean	The average value.
MRC	The Medical Research Council.
na	Not available, not applicable.
NDNS	The National Diet and Nutrition Survey.
NFS	National Food Survey. The National Food Survey was replaced by the Expenditure and Food Survey from 1 April 2001.
nlc	not low calorie.
No.	Number (of cases).
Non-manual social class	Respondents living in households where the household reference person was in an occupation ascribed to *Social Class I, II or III non-manual*.
NMES	*See* Non-milk extrinsic sugars.
Non-milk extrinsic sugars	Extrinsic sugars, except lactose in milk and milk products. Non-milk extrinsic sugars are considered to be a major contributor to the development of dental caries.
NSP	*See* Non-starch polysaccharides.
Non-starch polysaccharides	A measure of 'dietary fibre'.
ONS	Office for National Statistics.
PAF	Postcode Address File; the sampling frame for the survey.

Physical activity sample	Those respondents for whom a seven-day physical activity diary was obtained.
Plasma 25-hydroxyvitamin D; plasma 25-OHD	The biochemical index of vitamin D.
Portion	A portion of fruit or vegetables is equivalent to 80g consumed weight.
PSU	Primary Sampling Unit; for this survey, postcode sectors.
Quetelet index	*See* Body Mass Index.
Region	Based on the Standard regions and grouped as follows:

Scotland

Northern
North
Yorkshire and Humberside
North West

Central, South West and Wales
East Midlands
West Midlands
East Anglia
South West
Wales

London and South East
London
South East

The regions of England are as constituted after local government reorganisation on 1 April 1974. The regions as defined in terms of counties are listed in Chapter 2 of the Technical report (*see* http://www.food.gov.uk/science).

Responding sample	Respondents who completed the dietary interview and may/may not have co-operated with other components of the survey.
RNI	The Reference Nutrient Intake for protein or a vitamin or a mineral. An amount of the nutrient that is enough, or more than enough, for about 97% of the people in a group. If average intake of a group is at or above the RNI, then the risk of deficiency in the group is small.
SACN	The Scientific Advisory Committee on Nutrition.
se	Standard error. An indication of the reliability of an estimate of a population parameter, which is calculated by dividing the *standard deviation* of the estimate by the square root of the sample size.
Wave; Fieldwork wave	The 3-month period in which fieldwork was carried out.

Wave 1: July to September 2000
Wave 2: October to December 2000
Wave 3: January to March 2001
Wave 4: April to June 2001

WHO	World Health Organization.

Appendix G List of tables

Figures

4:   Nutritional status (physical measurements and blood analytes), blood pressure and physical activity

Tables

Appendix B: Response and weighting

Appendix D: Additional Food Consumption tables